HERE'S THE DEAL ABOUT

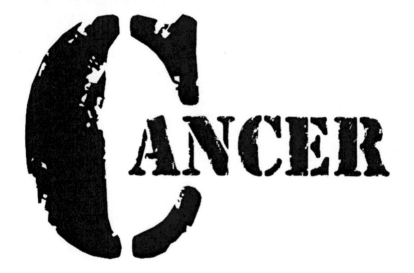

CANCER

Julie Mills
My personal story

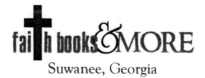

faith books & MORE
Suwanee, Georgia

Body of
Health
Healing from the inside out

1780 Oak Road
Suite A2
Snellville, GA 30078
bodyofhealthandlife.com

Ordering Information:
Quantity sales. Special discounts are available on quantity purchases by
corporations, associations, and others. For details, contact the publisher
at the address above.

Orders by U.S. trade bookstores and wholesalers. Please contact Ingram
Book Company: Tel: (800) 937-8000; Email: orders@ingrambook.com or
visit ipage.ingrambook.com.

Dedication

*This book is dedicated to Tommy's parents,
Milton and Sissy Mills, and his sister,
Mary Blount.*
*Thank you for your strong faith,
unconditional love, and for sharing such a
wonderful man with me!*

Foreword from Julie Mills

The material in this book is being presented in an effort to let the average person see that there are workable ways to deal with cancer. With conventional treatment, there is conflicting information and virtually no support for supplemental methods. I want to show you that it's all doable or, in other words, workable. I want you to understand that it isn't easy, by any stretch of the imagination, but it's simply doable.

You cannot incorporate supplemental treatments with the mentality of just "trying it." You have to take things seriously. It's important to build your immune function. In order to do this, you have to give your body vital nutrients on a daily basis.

By understanding how the therapies work, you can determine if they're right for your body. Once you decide on some therapies, how do you monitor them? You do that by understanding how they support your body's immune function. Ask yourself if they're reducing inflammation, reducing acidity, removing toxins, blocking tumor growth, providing antioxidants, inhibiting blood flow to the tumor (prohibiting growth), etc.

Once you're diagnosed with cancer, you have to understand that your body is broken. It's up to you to repair it and maintain it for life. This isn't the mind set of "just get the treatments over with and I'll be fine." The diagnosis of cancer is a wake-up call. A lifestyle change has to occur to keep the cancer from growing back. Your body already created an environment where the cancer can live. Without changes, it will continue to live. The incorporation of complementary therapies doesn't mean a person will survive forever. However, these therapies will improve a person's quality of life tremendously. Supporting your body will allow you to participate fully with the ones you love and in the things you love to do.

My family and I came up against some huge obstacles and many wake-up calls while battling brain cancer. I wouldn't wish cancer on my worst enemy; however, as I look around me, I see that it's an epidemic, but one that can be prevented in so many ways. There isn't just one thing that "causes" cancer. It's a cascade of many things that have gone wrong which means that there's not just one "cure" for cancer. A cure is the incorporation of many therapies that help fight the disease and keep it at bay.

You don't have to suffer so greatly while undergoing treatments either. If you educate yourself about your disease and your immune function, you can incorporate changes in your lifestyle and eating habits that can greatly improve your quality of life. As I said earlier, it's all doable if you just take it seriously. You have the rest of your life ahead of you. What are you waiting for?

I write this book to share my experience in the hope of sparing others the learning curve we had to endure. The unknown is the biggest fear factor. Hopefully, through my journey and what we discovered, you will -

- Have a light at the end of that tunnel.
- Be empowered with a plan.
- Have a direction when it seems as if there is none.
- Be able to make educated decisions instead of desperate choices that you later regret.

With warmest regards,

Julie Mills
Body of Health and Life, LLC
www.bodyofhealthandlife.com
julie@bodyofhealthandlife.com

Acknowledgements

I would like to acknowledge the enormous help given to me in creating this book. For their memories, their patience, and their guidance, I wish to thank my dad, John Davis, for his vision that my story would help others and his push for me to even do this book; Jon Watson, my best friend for life, for hearing and believing in me and bringing my words to life; and my kids, Mary Katherine, Eric, and Tony, for their patients and support while doing this project. I especially want to thank God, the Father, for instilling in my heart the passion and desire to reach out and help others who are suffering. Most of all, I want to thank Tommy, for living life to the fullest and being such an incredible role model to the world.

Table of Contents

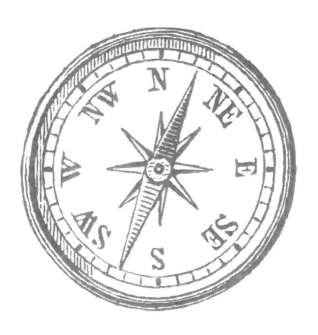

Chapter

ONE

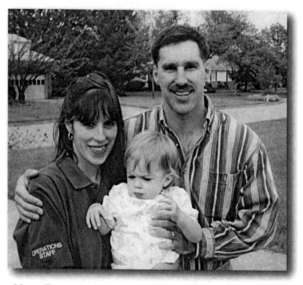

Mary, Tommy's sister; Anna, Tommy's niece; and Tommy
Day before brain surgery
April 1998

THIS IS MY STORY

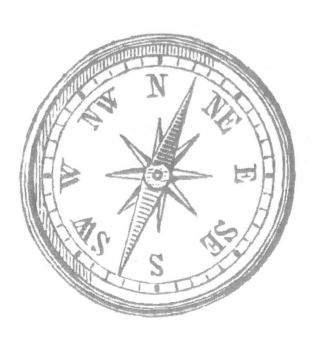

✐ I think it's the most important statistic of our time - cancer will take the life of one out of every five Americans. Believe me, I know. One of those was my husband of twenty years.

Do you ever find yourself thinking that cancer is a disease that only comes for the smoker? For the overweight? For the elderly? My husband, Tommy, was an athlete, a bodybuilder, and a Navy fighter pilot. As a F-14 pilot, he received complete physicals every three months. He was repeatedly assessed by Navy flight surgeons as being in excellent health. Then, in 1998, while on a routine flight, he experienced extreme tunnel vision and was barely able to get his jet and navigator safely on the ground.

We always thought we were a pretty typical family. Tommy had served 12 years in the Navy and had excelled in his field. We had three small children ages 7, 5, and 3. Tom was often deployed and I was a stay-at-home mom who somehow managed to be neck-deep in every one of her kids' activities. There was no time, or room, in our lives for sickness. And then - Tom started having headaches. At first, the doctors thought it was just a sinus infection and put him on antibiotics. After several months, however, he still wasn't feeling well. It was that final flight, when he experienced the tunnel vision, that started the wheels turning. A CAT scan was ordered immediately.

On April 16, 1998, I sat in stunned silence and listened as a doctor, whom I had never met, told me that my husband had a 9 cm, malignant tumor that was taking up a third of his brain. The doctor said that, due to the pressure it was causing, Tommy needed to have the tumor removed as soon as possible. We were scared. We were clueless. We were numb. And that's the state-of-mind we were in as we began making the most important decisions of our lives.

We asked for a second opinion and the scans were reviewed by another neurosurgeon. "Maybe this was all just a medical mistake", I kept telling myself. The doctor confirmed what we had been told and agreed that the tumor needed to be removed immediately. At the time, we didn't know that some surgeons and hospitals are better equipped than others to perform these types of complicated procedures. We just assumed we were in good hands and scheduled the surgery for the following Monday at 8:30 a.m.

My Diary

The Surgery

DAY 1

❧ Tommy's surgery lasted eight hours. They put him on a ventilator and gave him a drug to induce a coma in an effort to keep his brain inactive, which would help reduce the swelling. I was told the tumor was vascular which means it bled a lot during the operation and was quite a challenge for the surgeon. During the surgery, the pressure in Tom's head frequently went up to levels between 28 and 30. The normal pressure is

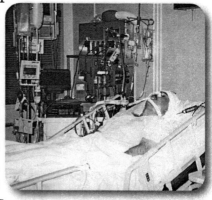

below 16. We were told before the surgery that, if it was bad and the tumor was a high malignancy, they would take enough out to get rid of Tommy's headaches but then close up early.

When the nurse came out sooner than she should have, we knew it wasn't a good report. It was touch and go that night as to whether Tommy would have to go back to surgery for another procedure to relieve the pressure in his brain. His body was literally covered with tubes and IV's. My heart pounded every time I looked at him. To help me focus and pass the time, I asked the nurse about each and every device that was hooked to him. I made it my job to monitor the instruments and to participate in his recovery rather than just sit there scared and helpless.

The nursing staff was great. They told me everything that was going on and thanked me for my help. I held Tommy's cold, limp, hand through the night and every time a nurse came into the room, I updated her on his progress. We made a great team.

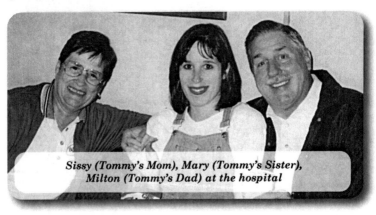

Sissy (Tommy's Mom), Mary (Tommy's Sister), Milton (Tommy's Dad) at the hospital

The whole family was out in the waiting room: Mary, Tommy's sister; Milton and Sissy, Tommy's parents; and my sister, Kathy. More would be flying in the next day. Some friends and other squadron wives were there, too. They were always right there for me anytime I stepped out of the room to stretch my legs.

DAY 2

❦ The outpouring of support I received was unbelievable! The rest of my family arrived bright and early. My parents, John and Judy, and my sister, Kim, all flew in along with my brother-in-law, Alan. Navy wives had been there all night and more came that morning. I can't tell you how overwhelmed I was to be surrounded by so many.

I was approached by the medical staff to sign a document that stated I had been informed there was a possibility that Tommy wouldn't live more than 72 hours. Those words crushed my heart. All of my decisions became urgent and I certainly didn't feel that I was in any frame of mind to be making them. It never occurred to me that Tommy might die from the surgery. I thought his brain might not be the same, but never that he could die. Not Tommy.

After the long, hard night, I spoke with the doctor again. The pressure in Tom's brain was still too

high, and I agreed to another surgery. I had helped monitor his condition through the night and knew it wasn't getting any better. This operation would remove more of the tumor plus the part of his brain that was already affected by the cancer.

I had to make the choice between Tommy possibly dying by stroke due to there being too much cranial pressure, or removing more of his brain and not having our old Tommy back. The frontal lobe area controlled personality and reasoning. Before, I really wanted Tommy back just the way he had been. Now, I just wanted him to be able to say goodbye to everyone in his own words and in his own way.

Tommy went back into surgery and more of the tumor was exposed and removed along with the damaged part of his brain. Afterward, the doctor told me that Tom should function no differently than he had in the past three months. I thought, "I can live with that." I was still scared and concerned about signs of brain damage. We wouldn't know anything until he woke up. He was stable, but still in a coma.

DAY 3

✿ I had a lot of people talking to me about a lot

of things - my future, Tom's medical retirement, insurance, and the Veterans Administration (VA). While I believed retirement was inevitable, it was very frustrating to try to sort through everything that was being thrown at me.

Taking care of the disability insurance and issues with the Medical Board was harder than I thought. I called Tommy's best friend and fellow pilot, John Owens, and asked if he could go with me and sit in on the meeting. I knew he would give me straight

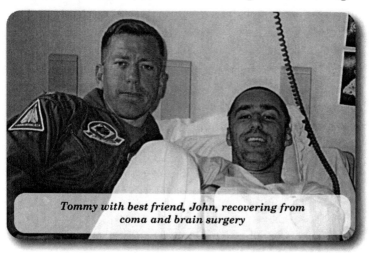

Tommy with best friend, John, recovering from coma and brain surgery

information and would advise me from a pilot's point of view. To sit in that office and have to sign Tommy's retirement papers was almost unbearable. Tommy loved flying. It was a huge part of who he was. I'd always assumed retiring from the Navy would, one day, be his decision, not mine. I just wanted him to wake up so he could make that decision and have some control over his life again. I was grateful for John's help and comfort, but it tore my heart out to bring an end to Tom's career.

Tommy was still in a coma. They had shaved his mustache so that the ventilator tube would fit more securely. I had never seen him without his mustache. It was disturbing to see him that way because he actually looked like a totally different person. Everything was changing so fast and it seemed my heart was sinking deeper by the minute.

They changed the wrapping on Tommy's head. The old one had been loose and stained with blood and medicine. He now looked cared for and clean. His body temperature was getting warmer. His hands had been ice cold due to lack of activity. Now there was more activity in the brain which was a sign he was trying to wake up.

I felt mentally and physically exhausted. There were so many visitors that they all but took over the waiting room. I felt as if I had to make conversation and be entertaining. Everyone had so many questions and I just didn't have answers. I had no clue what to do!

DAY 4

∽   Things became a little quieter. There were fewer people at the hospital. The stress about Tommy's cranial pressure lessened and there was no more pending surgery. Until then, I'd been on automatic pilot. I was constantly inundated with questions and had to make decisions with virtually no time to process things or comprehend the gravity of the situation. I finally had a little time to think when the hospital provided an apartment nearby. It brought a welcomed end to sleeping on the floor.

We finally learned Tommy's diagnosis - a high-grade, primary tumor called Anaplastic Oligodendroglioma. We were told it was a rare condition which accounted for only 4% of all brain tumors. According to the statistics, life expectancy was 2½ years. That news was hard to swallow. As you can imagine, I felt as if I had been hit by a train. Again! I was at my lowest and, now, there were even more decisions to be made. It seemed all my energy poured out onto the floor.

While I couldn't seem to think straight, I also didn't panic. I was just plain sad. We had been fighting for Tommy's short term survival and now we were going to have to fight for his extended life! He would need both chemotherapy and radiation and

I had absolutely no idea what was involved and what lay ahead.

I spoke to the rest of the family about the diagnosis. Pathology confirmed an Anaplastic Oligodendroglioma. I couldn't spell it or pronounce it and knew nothing about this type of tumor. I gave this information to friends and family and got a lot of information back. At that point, however, I was really having trouble concentrating on anything. When I tried to read something, I found myself reading the same sentence over and over before finally comprehending the information.

The doctors decided to take a CAT scan to see how much room there was for swelling in Tommy's brain. They would keep him sedated if the brain was being crowded. The less brain activity, the less swelling. Reduced swelling meant that they could reduce the sedative and try to wake him up.

During that procedure of reducing the sedative in an effort to wake Tommy, there were a lot of "medical" things going on. Tom was fighting the ventilator tube and his own body. There were multiple nurses working on him. They put things in IV's, moved him around, reset monitors, and requested procedures from other staff members. With all the activity going on around him, I had to just step back from Tom and let the medical team handle the immediate lifesaving measures. I felt so useless. I just hoped he wouldn't fight his body too much and would open his eyes. I didn't know what was happening and couldn't have done anything about it if I had.

I had to learn to get out of the way and trust the staff. That wasn't my nature. Tommy was usually deployed for six months at a time and, with three kids to raise, I was used to taking the bull by the horns! I knew, however, that I couldn't possibly understand the whole process. Things had to happen quickly and I needed to move aside and let the medical staff do their jobs.

I hadn't had any quiet time to sort things out. Finally, without any real cause, I exploded at my sister, Kathy. That ended up breaking the dam and letting the tears flow. We went back to the apartment and talked and cried and talked some more. I really needed that. She provided a safe, loving space for me to let everything go. So many people were asking what I wanted or needed, but I had no idea. I was getting so angry at people who felt sorry for me or had that sad look. I wanted people to visit, but I wanted them to talk about themselves and their outside lives and not dwell on the "poor Julie" thing. I also realized that all of this - the diagnosis of cancer, the urgency of the decisions, the life changing events, and the crisis situation - was completely foreign to me. How could they possibly think I knew what I wanted or what would help in the situation? I had a life-and-death situation on my hands. All eyes were on me and my brain was in neutral. I just needed people to step in and handle the kids, the house, the mail, the phone calls, the whatever. I didn't care about the details. I just needed it done.

DAY 5

❧ I was totally drained. I had a limited supply of clothing and had not fixed my hair in days. I missed my children. They seemed to be doing great, but Tony, my youngest, was only three years old and just wanted his mommy. I wanted to go home and hug them all, but there was no way I could leave Tommy. I had a wonderful support system with in-laws, parents, friends, and the Navy to help me. What I really wanted, though, was just to be with my kids.

I told the nursing staff my dilemma and they came back with a beeper. We came up with codes so that they could communicate with me about any changes and reach me in an emergency. "444" meant Tommy was waking up, "911" indicated an emergency, and "000" meant to just call in. I got to go home and spend some much-needed time with the kids. That night, I returned to the hospital rested and ready for Tommy to wake up.

The doctors were pleased with his progress and were very confident that he would come out of this thing. Tom didn't look good, but his hands were a lot warmer and I could feel more of a pulse in them. There was nothing for me to do except sit and wait.

DAY 6

It was Sunday and it seemed the whole world was praying for Tommy and our family. God must have been listening because, finally, Tommy came out of the coma and woke up! He began to respond to questions and everyone was so excited! If he could respond to questions, they could tell him what to do in order for them to remove the ventilator tube quickly and more easily. The ventilator was readjusted to see how he would do on a lower setting. If all went well, it could be removed.

When the ventilator tube came out, Tom started talking immediately. His words were muffled and slow at first, but got better. I was excited, and yet scared at the same time. My stomach sank when I heard the slowness of his speech. The first thing I thought was that he had suffered major brain damage. I had no idea at that point that the brain would need an extremely long time to heal.

I was so grateful that Tommy had pulled through the surgery, but I was also petrified that he would be disabled for the rest of his life. My heart ached for him. One of my biggest initial fears about the surgery was unfolding right in front of me. I wanted all of Tommy back, not just part of him. On the other hand, we were excited that he had his wits about him. He knew who we were and was rather demanding - excellent signs of progress! He was on the road to recovery!

DAY 7

∾ Tommy was moved from ICU to a private room on the oncology floor. We were all excited because he was hungry and began eating solid food. He constantly talked about his career. He hadn't grasped what had happened to him. The doctor explained to him that the tumor was malignant and that he needed further treatment. When it was just us in the room, he couldn't let go of his career as a pilot. Flying defined who he was. It was his life's dream. At that moment, no one was going to argue with him about flying. Lord knows, I was not going to tell him he was retired from the Navy.

Tommy thought the nurses and I were changing the settings on the machines to confuse him. He thought I was telling them to give him medications to keep him asleep. All of that broke my heart. All I could do was repeatedly assure him that it wasn't true and that I loved him. It amazed me to realize that people can hear when they're in a coma. They might get the facts mixed up, but they really can hear.

In spite of his confused state, all-in-all, Tom was improving by the hour. It would take awhile, however, for him to really get the big picture.

DAY 8

✍ I planned to let the kids see their daddy in the afternoon. I didn't know how they would react. Tommy had changed so much in the last week. They had shaved his head and mustache and he had lost 20 pounds. The staples had been removed from the incision, but the scar was still pretty scary. It went across the top of his head from one ear to the other. He had lost a lot of strength which made him appear frail; not the bodybuilder, fighter pilot daddy the kids were used to seeing.

When Mom brought the kids to the hospital, they couldn't go into the room since they were not old enough. So, I brought Tommy to the waiting room in a wheelchair. I could tell the kids were a little scared of all this. They weren't sure what to think about their daddy. They seemed shy and scared that they would hurt him if they touched him. We all stayed calm and loving. Tommy handled it well. We let them approach him on their own time.

Mom had helped them make cards. Showing Tommy their cards made it easier for the kids to get close to him. He let them climb in his lap and look at his scars. The visit was short but very good. It was important for them to process what had happened to him.

DAYS 9-12

Tommy continued to improve by the hour. We began to notice, however, that he was experiencing a lack of focus and wasn't very motivated. He didn't take initiative with things and struggled to stay on task. For example, it took him at least 30 minutes to brush his teeth. He went on and on with his stories and couldn't get to the point. His inhibitions were affected and he talked about sex a lot. The doctor said it would take time for him to relearn tactfulness.

We weren't too happy with what the oncologist had to say. Even though Tommy's tumor was a rare type, all they had to offer was standard treatment. There wasn't much documentation about the right treatment for his type of cancer. The doctor said the general rule of thumb was to be very aggressive in the beginning and to do the experimental trials if the cancer recurred.

Standard treatment for a rare tumor did not sit well with Mary, Tom's sister, or with me either. At that point, we started researching other options. Thankfully, instead of being shocked and overwhelmed, by that time, I was able to focus on looking for answers.

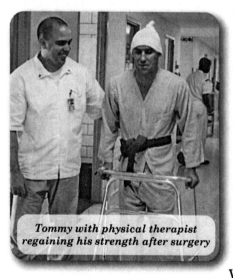

Tommy with physical therapist regaining his strength after surgery

We went on the Internet and to bookstores. We asked everyone we saw if they knew anyone who had a brain tumor. A friend of my sister-in-law told her about someone she knew that had a brain tumor. She had gone to a brain tumor center and had great success. We followed up with the information and found a specialist for neuro-oncology at Duke University Medical Center who treated brain tumors on a regular basis. We thanked God that we had asked the questions that led us to that discovery.

DAY 13

❧ It was May 2. We brought Tommy home. It had taken him two hours to get dressed due to getting sidetracked, talking on the phone, and eating. With help from Milton, Tommy's dad, I tried to keep him focused. It wasn't that he couldn't think what to do, he just had no motivation.

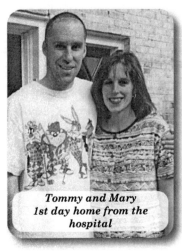

Tommy and Mary 1st day home from the hospital

Once home, he walked around the house and yard to check things out. We all took naps and then got up and got dressed for our daughter, Mary Katherine's, first communion. Tommy was able to attend and it was such a wonderful sight. Lots of people came up to us and hugged us. Tommy's presence warmed so many hearts. He held up well during the mass. Mary Katherine sat next to him the whole time. She was very proud of herself and of her daddy.

So much had happened over the past two weeks. Tommy and I were both so grateful to be sitting there at the communion. We wondered what was next for us. God answers prayer!

Here's the Deal:
Handle the News

✓ Take a notepad, or some type of recording device, when you're getting a lot of information so that you can go back at a later time and sort through everything you received.

✓ Get a business card from every person you talk to whether you think it's important or not. The insurance company will want to have all the information about every person involved with care.

✓ Take someone with you to important meetings to serve as a second set of ears in case you miss something.

Here's the Deal:
They Don't Know What to Do

✓ So many people don't know what to say or do in times of crisis. Really, nothing has to be said. Genuinely "being there" for someone is the best gift in the world.

✓ This is the first time this has ever happened to you. You probably can't answer a lot of questions and, you know what, that's okay.

✓ Make a list of your typical activities and daily chores such as feeding the dog, getting the mail, taking the trash to the curb, driving the children to school, preparing meals for the kids, doing laundry, mowing the grass, etc.

✓ When people ask how they can help, show them the list and let them "sign up" to take responsibility for a specific need for a specific period of time. You will have all their names and phone numbers on one document and will quickly be able to identify things that still need to be covered. This will relieve a great deal of stress for you and for those who want to help.

Here's the Deal: Ask Questions

✓ Ask the medical staff for clarification and explanation for everything that's happening so that you will feel more comfortable and reassured.

✓ The staff will tell you what's common and what's uncommon and will give you information about the steps they're taking and why. They'll tell you what numbers they're looking for on the monitors and what reactions they want from the patient.

✓ Ask the medical staff how long you can stay during in-room medical procedures. Ask them to let you know if they need you to step out. Keep the staff actively involved in helping you understand what is going on.

✓ By asking questions and becoming involved, you'll be an active participant in the recovery process. This lessens the fear and the unknown.

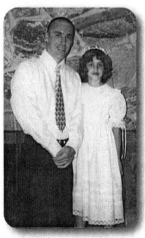

Tommy and Mary Katherine - First Communion

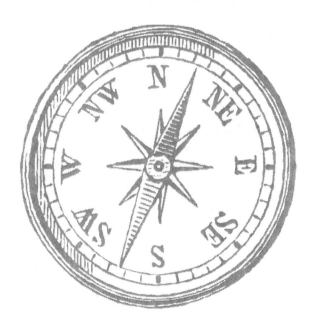

Chapter
TWO

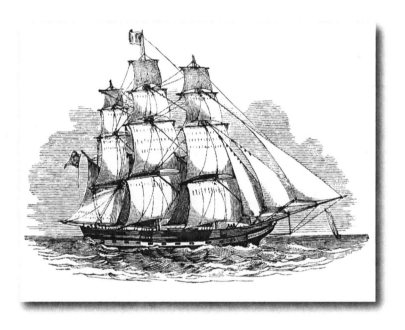

TREATMENT
DECISIONS

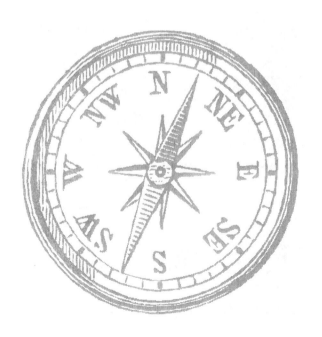

You're diagnosed with cancer . . .

✎ . . . and doctors tell you to do three things: surgery, radiation, and chemotherapy. They tell you that if you don't do them, you'll die. So, you say, "When do we get started?" Right?

Listen. Slow down and take at least a week to educate yourself on your diagnosis. It's important to empower yourself to help fight the disease. You have to educate yourself because the doctors can't do it alone. You are an integral part of the healing process. Don't expect someone else to do it for you.

In our case, Tommy was diagnosed on Thursday and had brain surgery on the following Monday. It happened so quickly that we didn't have time to think. The tumor had to come out! We didn't regret having the surgery, however, we did regret not researching surgeons. While Tommy survived the surgery, he had to endure much more stress on the brain than was necessary.

Tommy almost died and was then in a coma for six days. After talking to other brain surgery patients, we discovered a number of other methods that could have been used to decrease the swelling and lessen the time in a coma. I honestly believe the trauma was due to the surgeon's lack of experience with this type of brain tumor and the lack of advanced equipment available to the hospital that we had selected.

There are specialists in every field who know all the ins and outs of the disease and who have access to cutting-edge treatments that standard hospitals just don't have. Because networking between physicians is limited, your local doctor may not refer you to a specialist who is the most highly trained in caring for your specific diagnosis. The specialists you want are the ones writing the medical journals - not the ones reading them!

Because Tommy's tumor was rare - again, only 4% of all brain tumors - we weren't comfortable using "standard" treatment in our follow-up care plan. After much prayer and research, we found a wonderful hospital that specialized in brain tumors. I encourage you to find hospitals and surgeons that specialize in your type of cancer.

I'm sure your doctor is caring and is knowledgeable about a lot of things. However, he may not have a great deal of experience with your particular disease. He's doing his best. You're not hurting his feelings or questioning his abilities if you request a second opinion. It's about your care, not the feelings of the doctor.

You have to do the research yourself and request

that your records be sent for a second opinion. If the results are consistent, consider it validation that you're doing the right thing. If, however, there isn't a match, more research needs to be done. This is the time you may want to consider going to a specialist. Even if you have to travel to get to the doctors who have the most expertise with your particular diagnosis, it will be well worth your time and effort.

With more knowledge about your specific diagnosis, some of the fear you might be feeling will be reduced and you will be more empowered to make the necessary decisions. This is your life or the life of your loved one at stake. Go with your gut, not with your fear.

What's important to know is that you'll need to research several areas such as where the cancer is located in your body and the various therapies for that type of cancer.

Once you know where your cancer is located, begin to learn the following:

- What does the organ do?

- How vital is the organ to the overall function of the body?

- What organs are next to the affected area?

- Can the surrounding organs be infiltrated with the cancer or affected by swelling?

- Can the cancer metastasize or spread to other organs?

- How common is your type of cancer? Is it rare?

- How many cases have been successfully treated using the type of therapy being recommended?

- How toxic is the treatment to the area in which the cancer is located?

Tommy had a brain tumor, but where was it located? What functions did it affect? We pulled up the information on the Internet and printed out the diagrams that gave a good visual as to what we were dealing with which made it more workable for us.

Researching therapies might seem too medical, too hard to read, and grossly overwhelming. I was a finance major so medical jargon might as well have been a foreign language to me! I kept reading and, after a while, was able to pick out important information such as survival rates, side effects, trial length and access, and all the other "who, what, when, where, how, and why" questions. I highlighted this information and put it in a three-ring binder. That way, I could go back and look for similarities. For instance, some of the treatments were the latest and greatest, but had survival rates of between 12 to 18 months. That wasn't good enough for me. I knew I had to find something more long-term.

The purpose of gathering this type of information is so you will be able to identify the red flags. Knowing where the disease is located will help you know the side effects from organ dysfunction. Knowing the type of treatment will help you know the side effects of the therapy. You have to have these pieces of the puzzle in order to know, for example, when you've had too much chemotherapy or radiation. Then, it's time to discuss alternative plans with your doctor. Don't forget to always consider quality of life issues and how much treatment your particular body can handle.

Here's the Deal: Get a Second Opinion

✓ Ask for your medical records and send them to research hospitals.

✓ You won't hurt the doctor's feelings if you go somewhere else. It's about you and your treatment.

✓ Asking for a second opinion will either confirm what you're already doing, or it will reveal additional methods of treatment that were previously unknown to you.

Here's the Deal: Do the Research

✓ Highlight: survival rates, side effects, length of the trials, and where the trials were conducted.

   • Note that a phase 1 trial has very little data compared to a phase 4 trial.

✓ Compile all of the information into a three-ring binder.

- Look for common factors in the data you've gathered.

- What makes one trial more successful than another?

✓ Determine if the benefits outweigh the risks.

- Are the side effects worth it? (Does it cause stroke, liver failure, etc.?)

- Is the survival rate long enough? (Twelve months wasn't long enough for us.)

- Go for the less-toxic approach first. (Chemo accumulates in the body.)

Here's the Deal: Educate Yourself

✓ Know where your disease is located and the function of that organ. Can you live without it? Is it possible for the cancer to infiltrate the area around it? Can the cancer metastasize to other areas of the body?

✓ Know your treatment plan and all the side effects. This is important when getting a second opinion and comparing treatments.

✓ Ask your doctor questions. There are no dumb questions! You're new at this, so if something doesn't make sense, ask!

Chapter

THREE

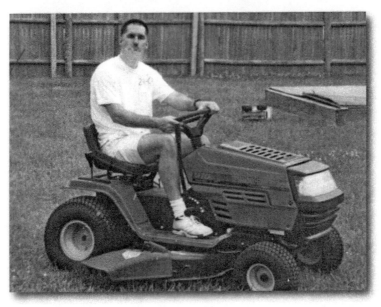

Tommy mowing the grass

THE NEW NORMAL

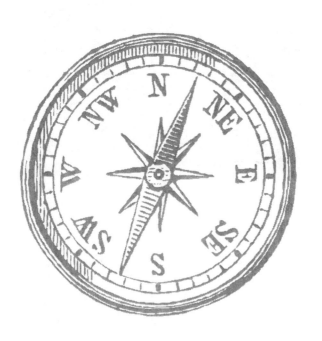

It had been a month since we left the hospital. We were so thankful that Tommy had pulled through the surgery and was able to come home. But, things were vastly different. We had numerous doctor visits, a lot of family staying with us, people visiting, food brought to the house, Tommy around all the time, and constant phone calls. Our life was far from what we had known as normal.

All of the new activity around the house took its toll on the kids. Our daughter, Mary Katherine, only seven, was the strong one. One day, however, without any warning, she hit her limit and started crying. Everything had built up and she was trying to let it all out. She ran out the door and around the block to a friend's house. We followed her, got her in the van, and we rode around and talked. She was so scared and didn't know what to do or how to interact with all the people coming in and out of the house. I told her she didn't have to "meet and greet" everyone that came by and that she could stay in her room if she wanted to. All she needed to do was love her daddy and be there for her brothers. That seemed to calm her and give her direction.

Eric, our five-year-old, middle child, was being very quiet. He went out of his way to please people and to help with his younger brother. He helped me by making his bed and getting dressed without me having to even ask him. He was being such a sweetheart and I wished I knew more of what was going on in that heart of his. I was always very careful to tell him how much I loved him and that he was doing a great job.

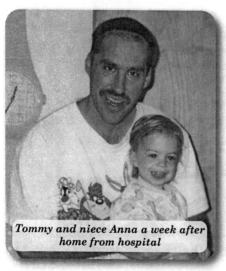

Tommy and niece Anna a week after home from hospital

Tony, our three-year-old, and the youngest, was not happy with all the changes. He whined a lot and was very hard to please. Being the youngest, he wanted Mommy to do everything - get him dressed, pick up his toys, and even feed him. He wouldn't let anyone else do anything for him. I realized this was his way of getting my attention. My heart broke for him but I knew I had to be there for Tommy and the rest of the family as well. All I could do was hold him a lot and give him all the love I could.

Tommy being around the house all the time created a lot of stress for me. Again, as a military wife, I was accustomed to him being away most of the time. The household duties and the kids had previously been my responsibilities. Now that he was home, he wanted to contribute to everything.

Having him question every little thing I did was unnerving. Sometimes, I had to leave the house for a few hours just to regain my sanity. I tried to always keep focused on the fact that we were fighting a malignant brain tumor. I was doing my best to give love and support to my children and husband and it was exhausting. I took on the job of medical coordinator and tried to manage all of Tom's treatments. It was overwhelming. I found that trying to respond to the outpouring of support from family and friends was nearly impossible. I literally could have used a secretary! There was only one of me and if it hadn't been for prayer and God's unfailing love, I don't know what I would have done!

⚬ Three months after we left the hospital, things were calming down quite a bit. Tommy had taken an oral round of chemotherapy. No IV made the treatment a lot more user-friendly. His blood counts were really good and he handled it well. There was a lot less activity around the house and no out-of-town guests. We tried a cancer support group but were disappointed with it. About 25 or 30 people sat in a big circle and talked. The general feeling was not good. We didn't hear or get what we were looking for. They were giving us more of a pep talk than help: "Hang in there. Take one day at a time." We were looking for specific information and a more-lighthearted atmosphere. We wanted people to talk straight to us about how they handled everyday life, but instead, we just got lots of hugs. Still, we decided that since the group, as a whole, was a good thing, we would keep meeting with them.

Each day, there was always something to be looked into or handled. It could be results of a scan, side effects of treatments, blood work to be taken, or benefits to be received. It might be physical therapy, people asking us to dinner, or a function for the kids. The days seemed to fly by. I had to make lists or things simply wouldn't get done.

Tommy took up a huge amount of my time. I had cut back on volunteering for things so that I could take him to appointments and hear what the doctors had to say. His physical well-being was good. I didn't have to take care of him, but I did have to drive him everywhere. We ate lunch together every day. Communicating with him was very important. I didn't want to lose my temper with him and letting him know my needs really helped us get through it all.

There was so much ahead for us to consider. I still felt overwhelmed. We didn't have to make any rash

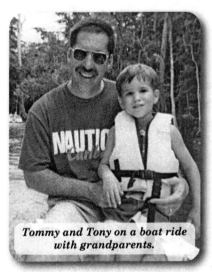

Tommy and Tony on a boat ride with grandparents.

decisions, but we had to figure out what Tommy wanted to do with his life. We talked about moving back to Atlanta to be closer to family. I worried about the whole cancer thing and if the chemotherapy and radiation would work. I didn't know what was permanently affected by the tumor and what expectations I should have for his healing. I was trying to run a "normal" household and the norm wasn't normal. My everyday life was so very different. I wasn't sure what my role was anymore.

✧ Four months into our journey, Tommy went to disability classes and got his board results. He was 100% TDRL or Temporary Disabled Retired List. We continued to look into our options. We would have liked to stay active duty through treatment and then retire. We also wanted to know if our insurance would cover the phase two protocol we were in post-active duty. We had a lot of people researching the regulations while we looked into VA benefits and Social Security. Dealing with the insurance side of the situation was another whole ball game. It was such an ordeal trying to figure out what was approved and not approved, what was authorized and not authorized, where to get referrals, and so forth. We now had a case manager so all I had to do was call one number when I needed something approved or if I had a question. That was a tremendous help.

≈ Five to six months after leaving the hospital, time had taken on a whole new meaning. My life went on with the busy task of being Mom to three little ones. I still had to plan the kids' birthday parties and summer activities. Basically, they were handling everything well, but they did little things that I knew were out of character. Eric cut his own hair one day and had been saying that he thought h e

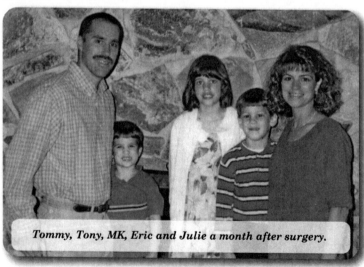

Tommy, Tony, MK, Eric and Julie a month after surgery.

was dumb and stupid. It broke my heart. But, he learned how to swim and he started riding his bike without training wheels. Tony was a little stinker. He loved bugging his brother and sister. He loved doing the opposite of what I told him. Mary Katherine was very emotional and seemed to be starving for attention. Although, there was a lot going on in her life, her prayers were so wonderful. She seemed to get the big picture a lot better than she let on. She was a smart cookie and I felt so proud of her.

I tried to keep the kids on their schedules with soccer, karate, dance, school, and church each week. I hoped that it would bring a little normalcy back into their lives. It was okay, by then, to leave Tommy by himself for long periods of time. He still couldn't drive, so I still took him wherever he needed to go. Out of town family and friends wanted us to visit them, and I planned trips and activities for us. Thank God for calendars!

We had to travel out of town to a different state to see Tommy's neuro-oncologist. Since he was able to take the chemo orally, it was mailed to our house. We had blood work done in town. Once a month, we traveled for follow-up visits. MRIs were done on base and then sent to the neuro-oncologist. I had become a manager, in some respects, and made sure appointments were scheduled, referrals were approved, scans were sent and received, and that we were ready to go for the next month. I'm telling you, it's a fulltime job.

Six months after Tom's surgery and diagnosis, his official retirement date was nearing. The squadron was giving him a retirement party. I

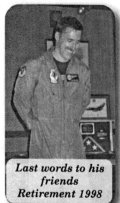

Last words to his friends
Retirement 1998

knew the coming days would be hard on him. He'd been a little down, and I knew the gravity of the situation had hit him. He realized he'd never fly for the Navy again. He explained to people that, "once they cut on your noodle, you can't yank and bank," meaning once you've had brain surgery, you can't fly. That was his fun way of being able to put into words that his love and passion in life had been taken away. We'd been talking a great deal about what he wanted to do next and we were very optimistic. I also knew, however, that a part of him was devastated because he couldn't get in that cockpit again. I felt so helpless. All I could do was be a sounding board and let

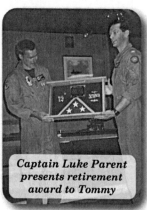

Captain Luke Parent presents retirement award to Tommy

him explore his options. As long as I managed the household and his treatments, I could give him the freedom to create a new dream.

We continued adjusting to a "new normal" and things seemed to be falling into place, but with cancer there were always "oh, by the way" things we hadn't encountered before. Experiencing blood clots and having to be hospitalized was one of many. The fear of infection at the site of the scar was another - not skin deep but down to the bone. The fact that Tom's immune system was suppressed was a really big deal. His blood count along with his ability to fight off infection, or sickness, was also a big deal. You don't want to get a cold. My reaction, when Tommy said he

Julie, Tommy, Tony and Eric at preschool event. Just a month after surgery.

had a headache, was almost comical. I would stop whatever I was doing and immediately ask him, "On a scale from 1 to 10, how bad is it?" Things with our health that we had previously taken for granted, now, meant serious jeopardy.

Tommy's tumor was located in the area of emotion, personality, and reasoning - aspects we had tended to take for granted. The doctors said they wouldn't know for another year whether those areas would be permanently affected. Tommy was definitely different, but his health was relatively good and I thanked God he was far from bedridden.

⊱ Another month passed. We asked the doctors what caused the cancer and the response was, "If we knew what caused it, we could create a cure. We just don't know." People had approached us about nutrition and lifestyle and we asked our doctors about this. They said, "Eat three square meals a day and live your life." Due to the fact that I was trying to establish a new norm and manage all the new challenges, researching nutrition therapy and lifestyle changes was too overwhelming for me. We just looked for Tommy to finish his treatments so we could go on with our lives.

⊱ It had been eight months since the surgery, and I began to struggle with forgetting things. I

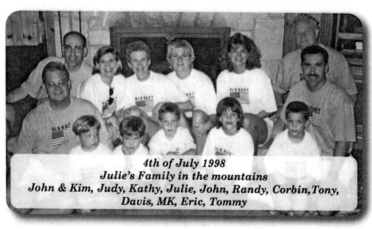

4th of July 1998
Julie's Family in the mountains
John & Kim, Judy, Kathy, Julie, John, Randy, Corbin, Tony, Davis, MK, Eric, Tommy

would write reminders and still forget stuff. I seemed to always be scrambling at the last minute. One day, I was supposed to have lunch with Eric at school. I got there right as lunch was over and he was so upset. I asked why he was so devastated and he said, when I didn't show up, he was worried something bad had happened to me. It hit me then how mad I was at this whole brain tumor situation. My six-year-old was afraid something had happened to his mother because she didn't make it to lunch! He just needed to be mad, not worried.

My concerns seemed so huge compared to a year ago. I used to be worried about getting my projects done, making it to the next meeting, or meeting the ship schedule.

Now, I worried about so many other things:

- My children being totally warped if Tommy and I didn't handle the situation right.

- Tommy's health as a life or death situation.

- Being a good wife and supporting him enough.

- Tommy not flying and the real effect that was having on him.

- Tommy's treatments and whether he would be permanently affected by the radiation.

- Starting over in Atlanta or wherever God would take us.

- Finances and being able to buy a house.

The list went on and on. What did God want me to do?

When I talked to a deacon at our church about these concerns, he assured me that the forgetfulness was due to stress. He said that's what stress does to you. In a state of being overwhelmed, you literally can't remember certain things. That made me feel a little better. He also reminded me that I was in God's hands and that He would give me the strength, focus, and the ability to handle all of those worries. I just needed to hand it all over to Him. Alone, I couldn't possibly handle it all. We prayed and I genuinely turned things over to God. I felt so much lighter and at peace.

As time went on, things were going pretty well. On December 3, Tommy had an MRI and we were told the scans were clear! Tommy was in REMISSION! We were so happy! But strangely enough, we were very guarded. We couldn't quite celebrate.

Here's the Deal: Let It Go

✓ Prioritize: Handle what is the most important and let the rest take care of itself.

✓ Change to a new schedule.

✓ Throw away the old calendar and make a new one.

✓ Don't beat yourself up. Just do what you can.

✓ When you find yourself the object of the patient's frustration, remember it isn't about you or the way you're handling things. It's the fear of the unknown that causes it.

✓ You can't always be in charge. Just be a good hugger!

Here's the Deal: Diffuse the Worry

✓ Ask for help. You'd be surprised how many people are just waiting for you to ask.

✓ Create a structure for your schedule.

- Keep a calendar.

- Make lists and put everything in writing.

- This is a team effort. Give everyone in the family a part.

✓ Pray. You can't do it all yourself.

- God will give you the strength and peace to deal with the new everyday life.

Here's the Deal: Create a New Beginning

✓ Let go of the old normal and create a new normal.

✓ Create a new dream together.

✓ Have new conversations about your new life (what really matters now).

✓ Hold onto, and only add, what will add value to your life.

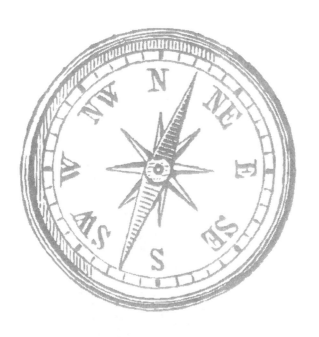

Chapter

FOUR

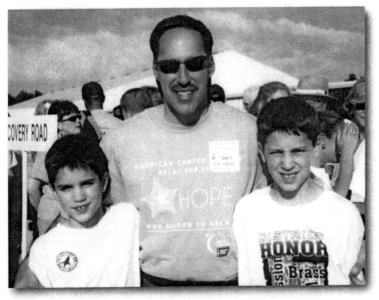

Tony, Tommy & Eric
Relay for Life 2004

IT'S NOT OVER

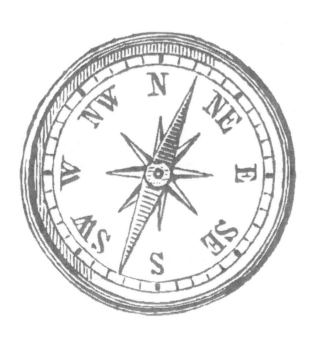

✑ Since Tommy and I wanted to move to Atlanta to be closer to family and friends, he put out his resume and got a job with the area telephone company. It was a far cry from what he had been doing in the Navy, but he was happy. It was amazing how much he had improved! Everyone said they couldn't even tell he had been sick. Life for us had certainly moved on. We had our house built a mile away from my sister, Kathy, twenty minutes from Tom's sister, Mary, and one hour from my parents. We were so excited.

Tommy had to have scans taken every three months. We adjusted to our new surroundings, schedule, and lifestyle very quickly. The children were in new schools and making new friends. We joined a new church and were very involved in the community.

With all the moving, getting the kids in school, and starting new careers, our lives were extremely stressful. We were a busy family with many activities. During that time, we did nothing to change the way we lived or what we ate. We were just trying to get to normal. While we weren't ready to incorporate changes, we did keep our ears and eyes open. For the next few years, we kept hearing more about alternative methods of treatment for cancer.

We asked our doctors over and over if there was something we should change in our diet or lifestyle or if there was anything we needed to be doing differently. We wanted to know what caused the tumor. We got the same answer as before - they didn't know, and if they did, they would cure everyone. They said to eat three square meals a day and live our lives. We did just that.

Tommy was working twelve-hour days and I was always on the run with the kids. There was no time to incorporate anything new into our lives. Who knew if a diet change would even help us? There was too much controversy surrounding the data. So, for the next three years, while Tommy was in remission, we made no changes to our diet or lifestyle.

We eventually moved across town closer to Tommy's work and to a less-congested part of town. A month later, in May 2003, Tommy had a follow-up scan. It revealed that the tumor had come back. In fact, they appeared in multiple sites. One was located in the speech area, one in the pons, or brain stem, and one was in the mid brain - the area between the two hemispheres at the top of the brain. Because of the multiple sites, surgery was not an option. The doctors felt that Tommy would respond well to the same type of chemo he had received before, so we went ahead with chemotherapy for nine months.

During those nine months, we did our research and started asking more questions about alternative and complementary therapies. The doctors kept saying they'd rather we didn't incorporate other therapies since they didn't know how they would interact with the chemotherapy. We listened to our doctors and didn't do anything against their wishes.

During that time, the chemotherapy stopped working. It became very clear that radiation and chemotherapy were not long-term solutions. They were little more than Band-Aids to us.

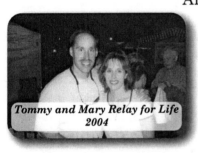

After the chemotherapy lost its effectiveness, our doctors offered very few options. They said we would have to wait four weeks if we chose to start a new protocol. After that meeting, we didn't feel comfortable waiting or flying blindly with a new protocol.

Tommy and Mary Relay for Life 2004

Mary and I had been researching alternative medicine. We decided to see a holistic doctor in Atlanta to discuss alternative therapies. The tumors were growing fast and we didn't have time on our side. The traditional therapies that we were being offered were just too slow. We needed to act fast and do multiple therapies at one time. The holistic doctor confirmed our philosophy that Tommy needed to be detoxed and his immune system boosted in order to get rid of the cancer or at least weaken the tumor and make it more susceptible to chemo.

We ended up looking outside the country for help. My sister, Kim, told us about a clinic in Mexico that her friend had gone to for her breast cancer. We looked into it and made some phone calls and discovered that we could get multiple therapies in a short amount of time. We decided to go for it!

I experienced a roller coaster of fear, anxiety, love, frustration, knowledge, hope, let down, confusion, prayer, searching, sadness, worry - you name it. I had to take deep breaths frequently. If it hadn't been for the support of family, I wouldn't have known what to do. It was reassuring to have them as my sounding board. It was also a load off my mind that Tommy was open to the idea of alternative therapy.

Our focus this time around was on Tom's quality of life. I'm talking about feeling good and functioning normally instead of being extremely sick or bedridden. Making the most of life is so very important when you've been diagnosed with a terminal disease. That's why it's so important to educate yourself and to be a part of the fight.

A friend of our family was diagnosed with stomach cancer. He went through chemo and radiation. After he passed away his wife discovered that there was no effective chemotherapy available for his type of stomach cancer. He was given chemo because that was all the doctors could offer. Had she known the facts, they could have decided to say no to that approach and seek other less toxic types of treatment. He would have had a much better quality of life and would have saved a tremendous amount of time and money.

Because of the experience of our friend, we were motivated to look for alternative forms of treatment. We wanted Tommy to participate fully in life. We didn't want the medications to impair that ability. We were struggling to find solutions, but kept searching for information. We were willing to turn over every stone in order to find ways to insure Tommy's quality of life.

Looking at the big picture, I realized the medical community was trained on illness and prescription drugs versus whole body wellness and natural ways of healing. In addition, doctors specialized in treating different areas of the body. Their job was to help those specific areas in which they were trained. In Tommy's case, they were looking to get rid of the tumor in the brain. However, in doing so, there was a risk that the medications might cause brain damage, liver damage, kidney failure, or a stroke. The medical community worked by diagnosing disease and then treating it with surgery, radiation, and chemo. It seemed to me that the impact of the medications on the whole body was viewed as a secondary or distant consideration. The bottom line was that doctors were just not trained in whole-body, immune-boosting health.

Most physicians discourage the use of alternative methods because they don't know how they will affect their patients' medications. Since complementary medicine isn't mainstream, the full understanding of its use is limited. Keep in mind that just because there's uncertainty, it doesn't mean you can't incorporate the therapies. If there is documented research that shows the supplement or complementary methods interfere with the medications in use, by all means,don't use them. Use your common sense!

Here's the Deal:
It Does Matter

✓ Your diet and lifestyle impact your overall health.

✓ Quality of life is important.

✓ Be involved in your care and keep researching.

Here's the Deal:
They Don't Have
All the Answers

✓ Doctors are specialists and focus on specific areas of the body, not the whole body.

✓ There is uncertainty about the effects of natural therapies with the medications.

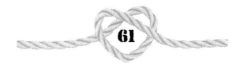

✓ Use common sense and determine if the therapies you want to incorporate are safe.

✓ Just because there is little documentation about a therapy doesn't mean you have to eliminate it.

Here's the Deal: It's Up to You

✓ Be an advocate for your own health.

✓ Educate yourself on natural therapies that will improve quality of life.

✓ Be persistent and stand up for your own health.

Chapter

FIVE

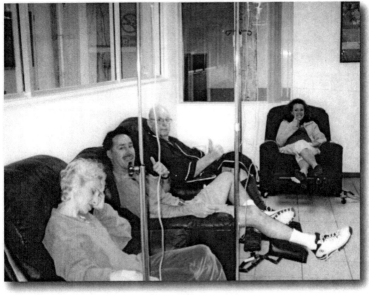

2004
Mexico: One of many treatments

EXPLORING NEW
OPTIONS

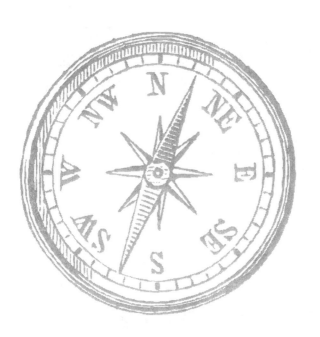

How We Even Got Here

After doing our preliminary research, Mexico seemed to be the answer to our prayers. Mary and I had put our nose to the grindstone and had researched several alternative therapies. We stayed with the ones that scientifically made sense and had been proven over and over. When we looked at alternative treatments, we began to see a pattern and understood more clearly how the body worked. We began to realize the importance of the immune system and expanded our trust and belief in the body's ability to correct the problem. All of this was very consistent with what was being offered at the clinic in Rosarito, Mexico.

We soon found that while most of the therapies we were looking into were not FDA approved, they had been sufficiently documented and proven in other countries. This obviously concerned us. We learned that the FDA's function was to oversee safety and application of food and drugs - not alternative therapies. Natural, organic treatments can't be patented because they're natural substances. This creates two problems. First, most companies do not fund the research. Why would they want to pour money into research for a substance they can't patent or have the rights to sell at a much higher price? Secondly, the procedure focuses disproportionately on specific results (required by the FDA) rather than whole body effect. Because natural alternative treatments help the whole body and are catalysts for healing, there isn't a specific, targeted result. In other words, chemotherapy, for example, kills cancer cells (and every other cell) and can therefore be documented and approved. Green tea, on the other hand, has many healing properties, but not one specific function and therefore can't be documented or subsequently approved. Once we understood this, we became much more open to the therapies.

Our plan was for Tommy to detoxify and build his immune system in order to fight the cancer. This seemed to be a long-term solution instead of a short-term "fix". If this didn't work, we had decided that we would set up a time with the oncologist and do the protocol that he suggested. I was keeping my fingers crossed that we wouldn't have to do that. We had high hopes and great attitudes!

Mexico

MARCH 29, 2004

Tommy and I flew down to San Diego, California. We were picked up at the airport by a member of the clinic's staff. Other patients arrived as well. They took us all to the clinic's office in San

Diego. There, we did the paperwork needed to check in. Then, they drove us across the border to Rosarito, Mexico. It was about an hour's drive to the facility which was located right on the beach! The staff was extremely friendly and informative. The facility was an older, two-story building, but was spotlessly clean. The guest rooms were on the second floor with the treatment rooms on the main level along with the kitchen and lounge areas. It had a pool and walkways that led to the beach.

It was still a little unreal that we were even there. After a lot of research, phone calls, and endless prayer, we had decided to go for it. We hoped we could build Tommy's immune system enough for him to take a different type of chemotherapy. We wanted him at his strongest and healthiest before the doctors began the treatments.

After dinner and a pep talk from the staff, I slept and slept and slept. I was finally relaxing and my stiff neck was gone. The clinic offered a detox program for companions. It sounded awesome, so I decided to do it.

There were so many different types of therapies and the medical staff was well-trained. They took every precaution with each individual. They were much more professional than I had expected. It amazed me that those therapies weren't offered in the US. They did no harm, only good, and the healing was tremendous.

MARCH 30, 2004

Tommy was hooked up to an IV that dripped all day. He rolled his IV pole around wherever he needed to go. One bag contained hydrogen peroxide, another chelation, and still another

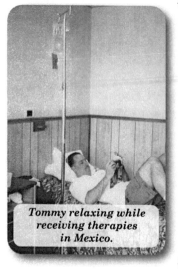

Tommy relaxing while receiving therapies in Mexico.

vitamins. He also had a physical including blood work, a chest x-ray, ultrasounds of the abdomen, and an EKG.

We were then introduced to the Mag Ray Heat Lamp, a specially-designed device placed over the tumor that magnified the effectiveness of deep-penetrating infrared heat. Unlike other heat lamps, it penetrates deeper and has a longer-lasting effect, but is much safer than any type of radiation. Good cells dissipate the heat evenly and bad cells die. Tommy used it to reduce swelling and to heat up the tumor to help weaken the cancer cells and to make them vulnerable to therapy.

We also utilized the Rife machine. This device works through frequencies that specifically affect disease-causing microorganisms. The process causes cells of the microorganisms to lose their integrity. They are then more vulnerable which results in their destruction and the release of their cellular waste and toxins into the bloodstream. Electrodes are placed on the body at the site of the disease, on the hands, or under the feet. Once the Rife machine is turned on, the frequency waves travel through the body and destroy all cells affected by that frequency. Normal, healthy cells remain unaffected by the frequency levels specific to the targeted microorganisms.

Tommy received the Far Infrared Ray which is a wave of energy that is totally invisible to the naked eye and capable of penetrating deep into the human body. This light wave produces heat much like the sun. Its gentle, radiant heat can penetrate up to 3.5 inches beneath the skin. The light and heat therapy work to enhance health by improving micro blood circulation, increasing the delivery of oxygen and nutrients in the blood cell, enhancing white blood cell function, removing accumulated toxins by improved lymph circulation, and much more.

Oxygen is a nontoxic, effective therapy that suffocates cancer cells. Healthy cells get their energy from oxygen. Cancer cells get their energy from sugar and other sources. High doses of oxygen actually suffocate cancer cells. To get the high doses of oxygen that are needed for effective therapy, a hyperbaric chamber is used. Tommy went inside an enclosed tube which was infused with O3 molecules which gave extra oxygen to his cells. He always felt energetic after the hyperbaric treatments.

He liked all of the different therapies. Each of them was very tolerable with absolutely no pain. Tom was feeling much better and we were learning so much about the body.

We met with the doctor that runs the clinic. He could only come there one day a week by U.S. law. He said that the therapies worked on the brain because the blood/brain barrier accepted natural things such as oxygen, enzymes, protein, and so forth. The blood/brain barrier is a problem when trying to administer chemo because the chemicals are foreign, not natural, and the brain fights their acceptance. He said that he has had the best results with brain cancer in children.

We asked about diet because we were surprised that they served foods such as meat and butter. He said that we should cut out sugar, refined wheat, and fried foods. We had met people there who had done a lot of research in nutrition. We kept getting more information about diet.

We learned that the key is to decrease cancer's fuel supply - sugar! Cancer patients need a diet low on the glycemic index or GI. Things that have a high glycemic factor are major components in feeding cancer and breaking down the immune system. We also found that sugar doesn't have to be in the form of table sugar. The body converts carbohydrates into sugar.

The GI is a ranking of carbohydrates on a scale from 0 to 100 according to the extent to which they raise blood sugar levels after eating. Foods with a high GI are those that are rapidly digested and absorbed resulting in marked fluctuations in blood sugar levels. Low-GI foods, by virtue of their slow digestion and absorption, produce gradual rises in blood sugar and insulin levels. They have proven health benefits.

The doctor confirmed what Mary and I had discovered with our research. Traditional treatments are incredibly toxic and are not long-term solutions. The long-term solution is the strength of our body's immune function. We experience disease in our bodies because our immune system is broken, out of balance, and not functioning correctly. Now is the time to go the extra mile and change our lifestyles! When we do, we're giving ourselves a better quality of life and a second chance to live well and live long.

I was still having a hard time wrapping my brain around all the treatments Tom was receiving. I couldn't quite understand, for example, how ultraviolet rays could kill bad things through the skin. I decided that time would tell, and maybe, when I receive some of my treatments, I'd be more convinced. I knew the clinic would help; I just didn't understand all the procedures.

MARCH 31, 2004

Tommy started Insulin Potentiation Therapy (IPT) which would allow him to receive smaller amounts of chemotherapy. Cancer cells have high metabolic rates because they're growing and can only use glucose as an energy source. They have more insulin receptors on their surface and have a more-intense reaction to insulin than normal cells. Therefore, if the patient is given insulin, the blood glucose level will go down and the cancer cells will momentarily be starved. If both glucose and a chemotherapy drug are given while the cells are starved for glucose, the cancer cell membranes will open for glucose and for more of the chemotherapeutic agent. Under these conditions, a lower dose of chemotherapy would be as effective as a high dose.

Tommy got out of IPT treatment and was shaking and very hungry. The doctor said that next time, he would decrease Tom's insulin because his blood sugar level dropped too low which probably explained his shaking.

The schedule was fairly light for us, but the staff always seemed to grab you for something extra. The people there for treatment were loyal and committed. I felt a sense of anticipation and hope in all of the patients and a sense of confidence and certainty in the staff. I so hoped this would work. All of our days were full of different treatments. We literally went from one treatment to another. Tommy took a small amount of chemotherapy with the IPT sessions, but due to the very low dosage, he didn't have bad side effects as he would if he were exposed to the full dose.

I truly believed the place wasn't just out to take our money. Everything was included except MRIs and CAT scans. There were doctors and nurses there 24/7 providing excellent care. We had access to everything. All of our treatments, medications, and supplements were included along with our room and meals. If a patient wanted to add another treatment, they could do so at no charge. If they wanted to stay an additional week, they could stay at a minimal charge. None of the therapies were harmful, so I wondered why they were illegal in the United States.

APRIL 1, 2004

Mornings were foggy there. It usually cleared up, though, around two or three in the afternoon. The temperature stayed around 65°, so it could be a little chilly at times. As I said, the clinic was right on the ocean. The fresh, salty breeze was healing in and of itself. It was good to be away from home and all the hustle and bustle of daily life. We actually had the opportunity to rest. We were told rest was a key factor in the healing process.

We found ourselves sleeping a lot. When I asked the nurses about that, they said it was due to the detoxification of the body. It was common to get

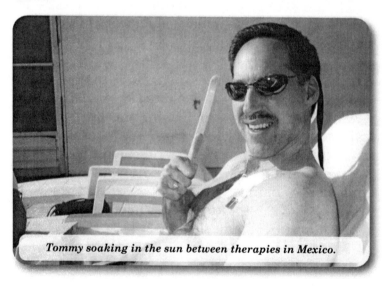

Tommy soaking in the sun between therapies in Mexico.

very tired and have flu-like symptoms because the body was working so hard to get rid of the toxins.

It was wonderful seeing other patients getting better. There was so much healing going on. A person who had a tumor-induced collapsed lung, was functioning well and the tumor was now gone! Another person with prostate cancer had arrived with a Prostate Specific Antigen (PSA) of 25. It dropped to the normal range, below 4, and then down to 1.5 with just dietary improvements! Another person came in with arthritis and was walking with a cane. He said that he had been in pain for 10 years. He had to quit his job and could barely get around. He was taking injections of some sort. He was now only on supplements and receiving one shot a month. He was almost as good as new! A man down the hall had pneumonia. He was out of bed, walking around, and looking great. We were fired up!

Tommy hoped to see the dentist about getting his fillings replaced due to mercury having been used in them. As you might imagine, mercury is very toxic. The cost in Mexico would be inexpensive compared to the states. They wanted him to have it done while he was doing chelation so it would draw any remaining mercury out of his body. He had a lot of fillings and I wondered how long it would take and how they planned on doing it.

We felt God had brought us there and we were hanging on for the ride. He had complete control. Everyone there had faith and trust, but also a little fear of the unknown. It seemed odd how the staff seemed so certain and confident. I guessed they had seen miracles happen many times. It was extremely difficult to think outside the box and realize what God could do.

APRIL 6, 2004

We got a shock! We had only been there a week and one of the patients we had become good friends with decided to go home and discontinue the therapies. I asked her if she knew something we didn't, like something illegal going on. Lots of things go through your head at a time like that. There's a tremendous amount of doubt when you step out of your comfort zone. She assured me that we were on the right path, but her situation had changed. Her blood counts were extremely low and she could not receive the IPT - one of the main reasons she had come. Her tumors were in her abdominal area. She could not digest solid foods well and the clinic did not offer juicing, so she was having a difficult time eating. She had gotten an MRI and learned her cancer had become a stage 4. Her last scan had been three months ago, and she had no idea the cancer had become so aggressive.

She didn't want her health to deteriorate to the point that she could not travel home. She encouraged us to stick it out and to follow the therapies at home. She had a great attitude, but realized her limitations.

I learned a lot from that event. Even though therapies are proven and working, sometimes, you have to step back and look at the big picture and ask yourself if it's the best thing for you. Often, it isn't. Sometimes, you have to just go home, regroup, and go with a different plan. Everyone has a different makeup, so not all things work for all people. That doesn't mean the treatments are wrong or a hoax; they may just not be right for that person.

The head of the clinic gave a lecture at lunch about cancer and its origins. He said that cancer is an ordinary cell that's deformed by a deficiency of vital nutrients in the body and an excess of toxins. This cell then mutates, or divides, instead of dying. By the time we're adults, all of our cells have stopped dividing. What the institute was trying to do was stop this division of the mutated cancer cells through the different therapies. If the cell didn't have an environment to grow, then it would die. I found that fascinating.

Tommy got the mercury fillings removed from his teeth. The dentist worked on one side of his mouth one evening and the other side the next. The

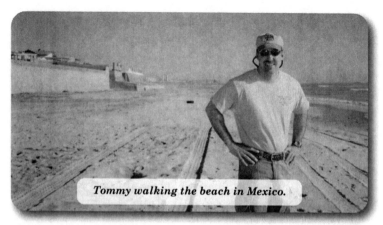

Tommy walking the beach in Mexico.

chelation drip Tom was receiving should remove the mercury from his body created by the dust. Chelation removes heavy metals. It's good to remove as many toxins as possible from the body so it can get to work on the cancer toxins.

We'd been there over a week. I was able to be quiet enough to get in touch with my feelings. We had been on the go so much that I hadn't really been able to know my own struggles and opinions. I felt like I had to fight to get anything - authorizations, co-pays, appointments, treatments, understanding, love, acceptance. I had been fighting so long and so hard that I didn't know how to stop. I didn't really want to stop because I thought if I did, Tommy might die. Thank God for my sisters and Mary. I knew without a doubt that they loved and accepted me and somewhat understood. I struggled though. I had rocked the boat a lot by stepping out on a limb, changing treatments, and incorporating all the alternative aspects. I trusted that God was leading me and giving me strength, but sometimes I didn't trust that I was hearing Him clearly or always doing the right thing.

Things Have Changed!

APRIL 7, 2004

❧ Around 1:00 p.m., when Tommy got out of the hyperbaric chamber, he realized that he was having trouble with his speech. He couldn't come up with the words to form sentences. His speech was filled with gibberish. For example, he said "ander" a lot. He was even having trouble writing what he wanted to say.

We saw the doctor and expressed our concern. He said it was probably swelling due to the IPT therapy. That wasn't uncommon. He started Tommy on a drip. He lay down with a slight headache. I was so worried. I wondered if the tumor had grown. The doctors said that the speech area already had damaged tissue from the tumor, and was therefore more sensitive to swelling and treatment. He didn't believe it was tumor growth. Things worsened as the day went on. I got scared and called for the doctor. He came and checked Tommy's eyes. There was some swelling behind the left eye. His stomach was also hurting. The doctor told Tommy to squeeze his hand, but he didn't understand. Needless to say, I was in panic mode. At that point, they put him on a steroid to bring down the swelling. The doctor said it wasn't acute swelling because Tommy could swallow and he didn't have double vision or any numbness in the arms. I was praying a lot!

APRIL 8, 2004

Tommy got up and showered. He could carry on a broken conversation. He seemed to be doing much better, even laughing. We met with the doctor first thing and he ordered more of the steroid. He said that he would expect improvement within 24 to 72 hours.

Tommy said the treatments must be working if he had this reaction. He was confident he'd be okay. He just didn't want the kids to see him like that. I didn't either. It would scare them just as it had me. I had to be Tommy's interpreter. I followed him around to complete or clarify his sentences. I guess being together for 18 years helped with that.

APRIL 9, 2004

It was our last day at the clinic. I spent the

morning packing. The doctors weren't sure when Tommy needed to come back. It all depended on the scans we would have taken once we were back in Atlanta. We had our instructions for the protocol of supplements to take at home. When we were settled again, I would have to dive into the insurance handbook to see what was covered out of the therapies we had received. I had a lot of work ahead of me.

I was ready to get home. I really missed the kids and my own bed. I was excited about improving our diet and lifestyle. It would be a challenge and an education process, but well worth it. Tommy was back to normal. He could remember his prayers and carry on a conversation. The doctors were right, it was just swelling. That little episode gave us a scare and a reality check! I thought this treatment would work. If the tumors were stable, we wouldn't have to do the protocol that the oncologist had suggested. We would wait one month and see from there. If the tumors were shrinking, we would continue with the supplements and nutrition. It was all a wait-and-see.

Coming Home

APRIL 10, 2004

It was extremely difficult to eat healthily while traveling. I never realized how unhealthy our foods were until I found out what was in them. We had been home only a few days and the reality of life had already set in. We were taking care of domestic life while trying to get on a supplement schedule. Some of them had to be taken on an empty stomach and some with meals. Trying to do this while traveling, and then getting settled into a routine at home, was quite a challenge.

At our son's school bus stop, a neighbor told me about her friend's husband who had a brain tumor and had taken a supplement called Protocel. I had never heard of it. I asked for more information and was open to learning about it. She called me that afternoon and gave me her friend's number. I called her immediately. Her story was so compelling that I ordered Protocel right away. Then, I looked up more information about it on the Internet and was intrigued. The major drawback to Protocel was that you could not use it with any oxygen therapies or several of the supplements the Mexico clinic had prescribed. It was designed to lower the energy of the cells, not raise it. So, we held off on taking the Protocel.

After Tommy's MRI, the oncologist called and said it did not look good. The tumor in the speech area was completely highlighted and active again and the tumor in the pons was larger as well. Needless to say, this news was a kick in the stomach. At first, I was mad, and then scared. I then started second-guessing myself. I finally just broke down and cried. We didn't have time to figure out what was right or wrong. I felt responsible for Tommy and that scared me. I was angry at the doctors and the politics of medicine. I felt like I couldn't trust anyone. Everyone had compelling stories - the oncologist, the clinic in Mexico, and my friend who used Protocel. Which way should I turn? I felt that chemo was short-term and I didn't want to accept that. I was tired of reading and trying to interpret all the medical jargon and struggling with how a stupid cell worked! I felt like I couldn't make another decision.

Each chemo treatment we did was a trial due to the fact that Tommy had a rare tumor. To be able to participate in the trial, he had to meet certain parameters such as size of the tumor, primary vs. recurrent tumor, male vs. female, etc. We called our neuro-oncologist to get the details of what was needed to start the new protocol. They wanted blood and the amounts of chemo he took in Mexico. We faxed the information to them and, within an hour, got a call from our doctor saying that because he still had some chemo in his blood, we would have to wait four weeks before he could do the trial. They also wanted him to take a combination of prescription drugs as inhibitors for the tumors until we could start the trial. We decided not to take the prescription drugs, but to take supplements that the body could recognize instead.

We talked with the doctors in Mexico about the bad scans. We got some interesting information from them. Sometimes the highlighted area of the scans was swelling with some of the cancer cells in the swollen tissue. It might not all be cancer. They suggested a PET scan to see what was purely tumor and what was not. Before we started any kind of chemo, we would request a PET scan.

Interestingly enough, due to the knowledge we had gained by our experience in Mexico, we actually had a clear picture of what was happening. We knew part of the "growth" the doctors were seeing was swelling. Tom had speech issues again, and had to take steroids to bring the swelling under control. The alternative treatments were working. But instead of creating an environment where the cancer could not grow, they did the opposite. For some odd reason, the cancer liked the oxygen and boosting of the energy to the cells. Normally, this would suffocate cancer cells, but not in Tommy's case. Now, we knew we needed to do the opposite. We had four weeks to make that happen. If not for the education on how the body works and what forms a cancer cell, we would have been totally devastated and unable to take another course of action. I had already done the research on Protocel and had ordered it, so we had it on hand. Basically,

Protocel is a chemical substance that, if taken on a consistent basis, lowers the energy of the cells. Due to the fact that cancer cells have lower energy than healthy cells, they're more vulnerable to the decrease in cellular energy. Healthy cells aren't affected by this decrease of energy, but cancer cells can't survive and will die. You can find out more about Protocel in the book, *"Outsmart Your Cancer"*, by Tanya Pierce. I actually spoke with her personally to get more details about Protocel and brain tumors.

We cut out the oxygen therapies and supplements that increased energy and started the Protocel. Through our prior research, we had found resources that could provide us with information about the plant derivative of prescribed drugs. So, the Protocel we decided to use was composed of plant supplements instead of prescription drugs. Why not give the body something it recognizes to help fight the tumors rather than a chemical that's invasive and has multiple side effects? Our source for this information came from Life Extensions and our Natural Solutions nutritionist.

Knowing how important it was to get nutrients to the cells, we continued on a strict whole food diet. This took a lot of planning and prep work. However, I was surprised at how workable it was. Just a little planning and a little extra cooking and the whole family was eating great and feeling great. It took me longer in the grocery store because I was reading labels. Once I found brands that consistently used wholesome ingredients, however, it became much easier. I was pleased that it didn't cost a great deal more. Cutting back on meats and increasing fruits and vegetables seemed to even things out. I had to go grocery shopping more often because, when you get foods with no preservatives, they go bad more quickly. Rearranging my schedule was a challenge, but I looked at it like joining the gym. It's difficult to work in at first but, once you get a routine, it's easy.

Tommy went back to work and was feeling great. With such aggressive, active tumors, how was he feeling so good? He was doing yard work and playing golf. It had to be the diet and supplements. They made all the difference. We were truly experiencing quality of life.

Here's the Deal: Chemo Is a Short-Term Fix!

✓ Chemotherapy is a short-lived therapy that creates toxins in the body and lowers immunity.

✓ Recurring cancer cells are more resistant to chemotherapy.

✓ The statistics for survival with chemotherapy ALONE are low (less than 10% survival rate).

Here's the Deal: You Have More Options

✓ Just because your cancer isn't responding doesn't mean the fight is over.

✓ There are other, less-toxic ways to treat cancer besides conventional drugs.

✓ Doctors aren't experienced or trained in natural therapies. Therefore, they aren't allowed to give them as options. Natural therapies are outside their scope of practice.

Here's the Deal: Think Outside the Box

✓ It's scary to go out of the norm and try other treatments.

✓ In order to lessen the fear of the unknown, get

more knowledge about how the treatments work.

✓ Understand on a cellular level what the therapy is designed to do.

✓ It's up to you to incorporate lifestyle changes. The medical system doesn't offer this type of therapy.

Chapter
SIX

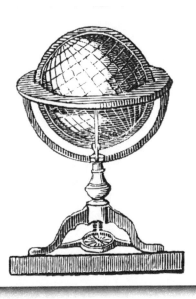

Eye Opening
Information

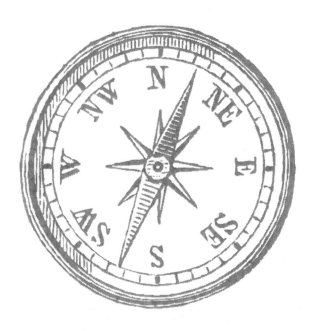

You Can Create an Environment where Cancer Cells Cannot Live or Thrive!

Before I talk about cancer-promoting environments within the body, I want to introduce you to Dr. Otto Warburg. He is a world-renowned scientist as well as a Nobel Prize winner.

Otto Warburg and the Anaerobic Cancer Cell

Otto Warburg, a German biochemist, discovered that oxygen-deficient cells ferment, or contribute, to the cancer process. The single root cause of cancer is lack of oxygen in the cell.

✍ Anaerobic cells (those without oxygen) become cancerous as opposed to healthy cells which are aerobic (those with oxygen). Dr. Warburg discovered that cancer cells do not use oxygen as their primary source of energy. The fact that a cancer cell does not use oxygen for energy makes them very different than normal, healthy cells. You must understand that an aerobic cell meets its energy needs through the use of oxygen. An anaerobic cell, on the other hand, is abnormal and meets its energy needs through other sources such as sugar.

Dr. Warburg's research is the basis for most of today's alternative and natural therapies. As part of his work, he discovered that cancer cells thrive in certain biological environments. These environments are lacking in nutrition, are oxygen-deprived, and are overloaded with oxidation and stress. His experiments have proven repeatedly that it is, in fact, possible to create an environment that prevents cancer growth. Even if a toxic environment has been constructed, lifestyle modifications can recreate these platforms and slow, or even stop, cancer growth. This discovery alone should give great hope to anyone who is suffering from any degenerative disease!

✐ In this next section, I am going to explain the cancer-promoting environment and discuss the role of proper nutrition and other positive personal factors. Please note that I am not a scientist or doctor. My explanations are intentionally simple and do not include in-depth medical details. I encourage you to do more research to fill in the gaps. The exciting part about this information is that it is completely "doable"! It might sound like a lot to take in, but once you change to a "whole food" diet, you have done over half the work! While it is important to educate yourself on why you are eating certain foods, don't get stressed out over calorie counts, portion sizes, etc. You are looking mainly for nutrient value.

I love sharing this information because it is so workable with any lifestyle. However, it does require consistency. This is not about "trying" it. It is about lifestyle change. You have to nourish your body on a daily basis. Consider food as your medicine. It is literally up to you to incorporate this vital part of the treatment, so educate yourself on what you are doing and why. Otherwise, it will have no value to you.

Now, take just a moment and look at your current lifestyle. How stressful is it? How healthy is it? Are you eating your fruits and vegetables? Are you getting enough oxygen? Does this example sound familiar?

You are young and work extremely long hours. You also travel a lot. Cooking is not a top priority for you, so you eat out...often! Your doctor says nothing about nutrition and you really don't go to him regularly anyway. You love coffee first thing in the morning. You're looking for some type of release, so you decide to take up smoking or a nightly glass of wine. Or three. You decide to drink sodas or energy drinks to give you a little pick-me-up at work, and water is not part of your day. You only get five to six hours of sleep each night, but you hit the gym almost daily. If you are a parent, throw the stress of kids into the mix and things are completely crazy. What you have done is created a perfect environment for cancer!

Remember, you don't just "get" cancer. It is the result of the breakdown of the immune system due to years of unhealthy lifestyle. Even though my husband looked like the picture of health on the outside, on the inside, the integrity of his cells was compromised. His lifestyle created an environment for disease and his immune system could not do its job. He had an immune system breakdown and, as a result, experienced a brain tumor.

Tommy's lifestyle was somewhat like this: He was a "meat and potatoes" kind of guy (very little nutrition and protein overload). He worked out every day - the heavier the weights the better - creating increased oxidative stress. He flew F-14s and landed on aircraft carriers; stressful but exciting. His head was exposed to electromagnetic energy (EMF waves to the brain). He was exposed to ultraviolet rays from the cockpit and high altitudes. He got very little sleep, no chance for his body to recharge. Do you get the picture?

◈ There is no "one cause" of cancer or disease. Therefore, there is no one cure for cancer. In this section, I will review some of the things that work to produce an environment in which cancer can live. Consider these topics in your own life and adjust where necessary to produce an environment where cancer cells cannot live.

- Oxidative stress
- Nutrition
- Sugar (glycemic Index)
- Food enzymes
- Processed foods
- Inflammation (Omega 3s)
- Acidity of your body (pH balance)
- Hydration (water)
- Oxygen
- Toxins in the environment: EMF (Electromagnetic Fields)

OXIDATIVE STRESS

❧ Most disease is caused by oxidative stress. This is a result of your metabolism and is necessary to keep your body at 98.6°. Unfortunately, oxidative stress is also destructive. It causes your body to produce free radicals which are like sparks going off in your body, hitting your cells, and damaging them. On average, you can get up to 10,000 hits per cell per day! To protect your cells from this type of damage, you need antioxidants. Antioxidants can only be found in fruits and vegetables. They essentially form a shield around your cells to protect them from oxidative stress.

Technically, what is going on is that "the spark" is a loose electron trying to find a match from a good/healthy cell to neutralize it. This process causes damage to that healthy cell. Only fruits and vegetables have antioxidants, or extra electrons, to neutralize the oxidation. If you think of energy metabolism as an engine, you have sparks and smoke. Those sparks from the metabolism are what hit your cells daily. That is why it is so incredibly important to arm yourself and protect your cells with fruits and vegetables that neutralize that extra electron that creates an unhealthy effect. The smoke is the toxic by-product of oxidation. It accumulates in the body and overloads the lymph (immune) system. With a weak immune system, you are more susceptible to disease.

Eventually, without protection for the cells, DNA is damaged. When that happens, the cell mutates and you have degenerative disease and/or cancer.

Nature has provided us with a way to neutralize free radicals with the antioxidants found naturally in ripe, raw fruits and vegetables. Antioxidants are the primary way to protect your cells, and the body does not have the capacity to produce them on its own. You have to replenish your body on a daily basis with antioxidants in order to help your immune system and protect the integrity of the cells. Otherwise, the cells are vulnerable to destruction and cannot perform their functions. This causes disease to arise.

NUTRITION

ⅎ One of the biggest factors contributing to the development of disease is malnutrition. Americans are some of the most overfed, yet malnourished, people on the planet! The typical American diet is nutrient-deficient. We eat processed, fried, overcooked, refined, and denatured foods. Fruits and vegetables are either canned or cooked to death or even microwaved. Hamburgers, fries, hot dogs, chicken fingers, and mac and cheese are typical. Where is the live food in that type of diet? Where are the protective antioxidants? If we don't give the cells what they need to work correctly, they malfunction and weaken the body's ability to fight disease.

Unfortunately, our thought processes go something like this...

- If it doesn't make me feel bad after I eat it, then it's okay.
- If it is on the shelf it must be safe.
- I'm doing good as long as I feed the family and have warm food on the table.
- Why would manufacturers make it if it wasn't okay to eat?
- I have been eating like this all my life so I don't have to change.

Then you have a heart attack and blame it all on the family genes! Did you know that genes only account for about 5% of disease! The rest is purely due to diet and lifestyle. We are a society of affluence. We drive rather than walk wherever we want to go. We buy processed, packaged foods instead of growing our own. We eat at restaurants instead of cooking at home. We have the money, so we think nothing of spending it on convenience.

Take responsibility for what you become. Stop blaming everything else. It truly does make a difference what you eat and how you live your life.

Nutrition gives the cells what they need to do the job they are supposed to do. A variety of fruits and vegetables are important because the body has a variety of functions. Did you know that the human body is comprised of over 210 different types of cells? They are all busy doing their own thing - for example immune system, hormones, heart, lungs, and colon - they all have to work in synergy. If we don't give them what they need to work correctly, they become sluggish and are not able to work efficiently. They can then become dysfunctional and weaken the body's ability to fight disease.

The opposite of malnutrition is super-nutrition, or putting the most densely nutritious foods possible into the body each and every day. Some foods are more nutrient-dense than others. Nutrient-dense foods include green tea (rich in antioxidants), brewer's yeast (great source of B vitamins), wheat grass (rich in antioxidants), sprouts (blueprint of the whole plant), freshly ground flax seed (great source of omega 3), dark fruits and veggies (the darker the more nutritious), colorful produce (each color represents different phytonutrients), walnuts, almonds, and sunflower seeds, and the list goes on. A wonderful supplement to get 17 fruits, vegetables, and grains is Juice Plus. It is literally whole food in capsules! Do the research and get the most nutrition out of every bite.

If you eat only two or three times a day, wouldn't it make sense to consume as many nutrients as you can rather than giving your body empty, destructive foods? Make every meal count. Give your body what it is crying out for - nutrition, nutrition, nutrition!

SUGAR

When a cell mutates into cancer, it wants to feed on substances that healthy cells do not. A real favorite of cancer cells is sugar. Sugar is a huge component of feeding tumors - especially brain tumors.

This goes back to the discoveries of Otto Warburg. He showed that cancer cells do not use oxygen for energy. Instead, they get most of their energy through fermentation of sugar or "glycolysis." This statement and discovery is pivotal in understanding and maintaining an environment in which cancer cannot live. "Warburg adamantly believed that the 'prime cause' of cancer was the switching of cells from their normal respiration process in which they use oxygen for energy, to the very different respiration process in which they use the fermentation of glucose for energy." In other words, Warburg believed that cancer starts when normal cells transform from aerobic to anaerobic functioning.

Refined sugar is processed, bleached, and chemically

treated. It provides no nutrition to the body. Again, sugar feeds cancer! It has been proven to be addictive and increases appetite. The most harmful form of sugar is high fructose corn syrup. This is a man-made, denatured form of sugar that spikes insulin and is high on the glycemic index.

Now, just a word about the Glycemic Index (GI). This is a measurement that ranks foods by how they affect blood glucose levels. The index ranks foods according to carbohydrates and how fast they break down into sugar. There are good carbs and bad carbs. Not all carbohydrates act the same way. Some are quickly broken down in the body causing the blood glucose level to rise rapidly. That puts them high on the glycemic index. Eating a lot of foods high on the index can be detrimental to your health because it pushes your body to extremes. Fruit juices may rank high on the index. However, eating the whole fruits with the fiber would make them have a lower ranking. The rule of thumb is the darker the color, the lower the glycemic rating. Starchy foods (light color) are high, but high fiber foods are low.

Remember, cancer feeds on sugar and that does not mean just table sugar. High index foods feed your cancer. Try to stay away from them! There is a vast amount of information on the Internet about this subject, so please do your research. There are easy-to-read charts and lists, so it really is not difficult.

Large quantities of refined sugar depress the immune system for up to six hours. You can easily calculate the amount of sugar you are consuming by dividing by four. Four grams equal one teaspoon of sugar. Twenty teaspoons of sugar lower the immune system for up to six hours. A twenty-ounce coke has 68 grams of sugar which equal 17 teaspoons. Think about this: one soda at lunch diminishes your immune system for the rest of your day! And we wonder why we are so sick and catch everything. Look at what we are eating! Now take it a step further and realize that cancer cells love sugar. When a cancer patient drinks soda and eats cookies, the immune function is lowered and essentially promotes cancer! In addition, the tumor's growth is sustained by the sugar fuel.

Sugar can be listed under many names in processed foods - fructose, glucose, corn syrup, dextrose, etc. You will find these names listed several times on ingredient list. This is called "divide and conquer." Manufacturers divide up the sugar in the ingredients list because they don't want you to realize how much of it is in the product. If all the sugar in a product was listed together, it would easily appear as the first ingredient. Ingredients are listed by most prevalent first to least amount last. Therefore, if they divide up the listing of sugars, the product appears to have less.

Beware of artificial sweeteners. They are not on the menu! Say no to all artificial sweeteners. They are chemicals that the body can't process and they affect immune function. Aspartame is the most common and you should stay away from it. It is extremely harmful to your health!

Another source of sugar is bleached, enriched flour. Products containing this type of flour act as simple sugars in the body causing blood glucose levels to quickly rise and trigger insulin production. This activity in the body helps cancer grow. Stick with breads made from whole grains. The fiber and nutrients are there to assist the body, not take away from it. Sprouted grains are an excellent source of nutrition. You do not have to stick to wheat. You can use rolled oats, rye, and barley as well.

Unfortunately, when you're a person with cancer, you actually crave sugar. Realize it is the cancer cells craving sugar, not you. So, the more sugar you eat the more you feed the cancer. A good way to curb your craving is to eat low glycemic foods such as fruit. For chocolate lovers, try a piece of 75% dark chocolate or use powdered, unsweetened cocoa in foods. You get a great chocolate taste without all the sugar.

FOOD ENZYMES

✎ Okay, so we are continuing to talk about the immune system and its breakdown. Another important cause of immune breakdown is lack of live food enzymes. You only get these enzymes from whole foods, and that means fruits and vegetables. Not meat! The optimal materials our bodies need to produce life energy are nutrient-dense and enzyme-rich foods.

Enzymes are involved with every process in the body. They digest food and take nutrients from it to build muscles, nerves, and blood. They assist in storing sugar in the liver and muscles. They build phosphorus into bones and nerve tissues, and attach iron to red blood cells. Enzymes are so important that enzyme depletion eventually leads to aging, sickness, and death.

You will not find enzymes in foods that are in a bottle, box, or can. Cooking or processing food over 118° totally destroys the enzymes in it. Cooking also contributes to nutrient loss. Pasteurization, sterilization, radiation, freezing, and microwaving either render food enzymes inactive or alter their structure. So, just eat as many raw foods as possible. There are some fantastic recipe books and websites out there for raw foods.

PROCESSED FOODS

✍ We have considered nutrition by talking about whole foods and enzymes. It's true - you are what you eat. When food is processed, or denatured, it has no nutrients in it. Now let's talk about the pollutants and toxins we are exposed to in our food and what they do to the immune system and to the body.

Since the 1970s, two major things have happened to change Americans' eating habits and have contributed to the epidemic rise in diabetes, cancer, and heart disease. First, fast food chains have popped up on every corner and second, partially hydrogenated oil (trans fats) have been introduced into virtually all processed foods.

Fast food restaurants were introduced in the late 1960s. Americans loved their convenience and they quickly became the norm in the 1970s. Their menus have very little, if any, nutritional value. Many of them call themselves "value menus" but I promise you, they are of very little value to the body. These foods are fried and processed so the body cannot recognize them as nutrients. Therefore, they are stored in the colon where they weaken it and promote colon cancer - the number one cancer in America.

French fries are not a vegetable! When you fry foods they soak up bad oils and the heat kills the enzymes so you are just eating empty, useless calories. A hamburger is not a meal. Yes, it fills your stomach and curbs your hunger, but it has no nutrition in it at all. The bun is made with enriched, bleached flour which has been stripped of its nutrients (denatured). The meat is full of antibiotics and hormones from the cow. When you choose a combo at the drive-through the bad definitely outweighs the good.

Partially hydrogenated oils (trans fats) are produced when unsaturated oils are heated and combined with hydrogen molecules which converts them to solid form. As a result, a new category of fat is formed - trans-fatty acid. The reason for this process is that the food will not break down as quickly, will resist spoiling, and have a longer shelf life. As of 2006, trans fats weren't listed as fat on food labels. Many foods that contained trans fats were labeled as "healthy," "low in saturated fat," or "low in cholesterol." These fats appear in the ingredient list as "partially hydrogenated" oils.
Trans fats are especially harmful because they raise bad LDL cholesterol while lowering good HDL cholesterol. People can reduce their risk of heart disease by as much as 53% if they eliminate trans fats from their diet.

The most prevalent sources of trans fats in the average diet are cookies, crackers, and other commercial baked goods. Trans fats are very common ingredients in packaged foods so read labels carefully to identify them. In 2002, the Institute of Medicine, a branch of the National Academy of Sciences, stated that there is no safe amount of trans fat in the diet.

Manufacturers are allowed to say "no trans fat" if a product contains .5% or less per serving. This information is incredibly misleading especially when you know there is no safe amount.

Here's a partial list of health hazards from consuming trans fats:

- Lowers HDL (good) cholesterol
- Raises LDL (bad) cholesterol
- Raises total serum cholesterol by 20 to 30%
- Lowers efficiency of B-cell response
- Increases proliferation of T cells
- Increases blood insulin levels (Cancer loves this!)
- Causes changes in membrane fluidity and ability to transport nutrients across cell membranes
- Increases free radical activity (oxidative stress)
- Increases breast cancer risk (Women who have

higher stores of trans fats have 55% higher risk of developing breast cancer.)

- Increases risk of heart disease
- Increases risk of type II diabetes
- Decreases testosterone levels in males
- Decreases fertility in females

Partially hydrogenated oils, or trans fats, has been talked about, researched, and proven to be harmful to the body. It's a preservative to keep foods on the shelf, not to keep you healthy. The body can't recognize the altered, or denatured, oils. These oils can stay in your colon for up to 30 days, weakening the lining of your colon, and thereby weakening your immune system.

Your body is working hard to fight cancer. Why in the world would you put processed, unrecognizable food into your body to distract it from its primary job of fighting cancer? It is important to read food labels. Please read the ingredients section carefully and look for bleached, enriched flour, high fructose corn syrup, and partially hydrogenated oil.

When you have an illness, eliminating toxins from your food is an absolute must. The idea is to get your body in a state to be able to heal itself and stop the growth of the tumor or whatever is contributing to your sickness. If you create an environment where the tumor, or the illness, cannot grow, where you have a strong immune system, you have a better long-term chance of fighting the disease.

INFLAMMATION

∞   Inflammation also helps cancer grow. Inflammation happens in so many different ways. High salt intake, for example, can promote extra water activity in the cell. The cell retains water which creates inflammation. Another thing that causes inflammation is the imbalance between Omega-3 and Omega-6 fats. Saturated fats (animal fats) are the source of Omega-6 fats. The typical American diet includes too much saturated fat and too little Omega-3 unsaturated fat (from fish & nuts). When the ratio is uneven, inflammation occurs. The ratio should be one Omega 3 to four Omega 6s. However, the typical diet has a 1/25 ratio.

Good sources of Omega-3 fats include:
- fish oils
- olive oil
- flax seeds
- avocados
- almonds

It is so simple to balance this ratio by increasing

Omega-3 fats in the diet and cutting back on animal fats. We accumulate too much animal fat because the typical American diet assumes that meat is the entrée and vegetables are good side dishes. Actually, the vegetables should be the entrée and meat should be a side dish. The body reacts to the imbalance of these necessary fats by creating inflammation around the cells. This is an environment that cancer loves.

ALKALINE VS. ACIDIC

There are many books and resources available regarding alkalizing foods and how to alkalize the body. The bottom line is that if you don't drink water or eat enough fruits and vegetables on a regular basis, you are creating a more acidic environment in your body. Some fruits you might think are acidic such as oranges and lemons, once consumed, actually become more alkaline. That surprised me. I don't want to get too technical here, but it is the key to why we must have nutrition in our cells.

The pH of the body is so important. Basically, acid-forming foods such as sugars, saturated fats (animal), white breads, alcohol, and coffee are extremely toxic to the body. We need an alkaline environment which is produced with the consumption of fresh vegetables and essential fatty acids. When you talk about consuming or starting an alkaline diet, you are talking about foods and drink which have an alkaline effect on the body. It just so happens that the foods that contain alkaline minerals are all the foods we already know are good for us. These include low-sugar foods, fresh raw vegetables, nuts, and fruits.

There are pH kits and testing strips available on the Internet and in health food stores to test the acidity of your body. There are also charts and scales for alkalizing foods. The rule of thumb is that blood pH should be 7.35–7.45. A pH below 7.0 is acidic and above 7.0 is alkaline. Why is this relevant? Cancer loves an acid environment. When you make up your menu for the week, make sure to include alkalizing foods. It is as simple as that!

The body has several control mechanisms to keep it at its proper pH and some of those include getting rid of excess acid or base by-products through the lungs, saliva, and urine. When your body is sick in any way, the pH balance is disrupted. Many times, the body is trying to keep up with the extra acid being produced. Acids result from lack of oxygen, eating an imbalance of protein, the intake of carbohydrates, the consumption of other acid-producing foods, and cellular breakdown and the production of metabolic waste.

As we have discussed, fruits and vegetables contain antioxidants. They're the basis for super nutrition. They house the enzymes necessary for the body to repair tissue. They also help create an alkaline balance. The less acidic the body, the less likely cancer can live there. Along with water, eating raw fruits and vegetables is the key to treating chronic disease and maintaining good health.

WATER IS CRITICAL

✍ Water is an essential nutrient and a must for good health! About 70% of your body is made up of water. In order to keep your organs functioning properly, to flush out toxins, and to improve lymphatic circulation, you have to stay hydrated. Only water serves this function; not juice, not tea, or any other fluid. Adding anything to water (lemons, flavorings, etc.) will activate the digestive system. The stomach then releases digestive enzymes and gastric juices to break it down. The water, therefore, is not absorbed properly and you do not get the full nutritional benefit. It is simply water, water, and more water!

When you have already created an environment in which cancer can live, it is imperative that you drink a lot of water every day. What is "a lot"? A gallon a day is not too much! You are flushing out toxins, hydrating cells, carrying nutrients to them, and giving your body a pure, clean source of hydration. Other benefits of water consumption are as follows:

- Carries nutrients and oxygen to every cell in the body
- Helps control body temperature
- Contains electrolytes and major minerals (filtered water keeps minerals)
- Cleans the stomach and aids digestion
- Cleans the intestines and improves absorption of nutrients
- Removes toxins from the body

While it is important that you drink water, it is also important that the water be filtered. Water from the tap contains chlorine and that's something you don't need. Chlorine is added in order for water to arrive at your home bacteria-free. However, it is not good for your health to ingest it. It breaks down friendly bacteria and interferes with absorption of nutrients from food. It has been linked to an increased risk of colon, rectal, and bladder cancer.

Think of it this way. The water facilities deliver your water to you safely by adding chlorine and other chemicals. A loaf of bread is delivered safely to the store wrapped in a plastic bag. Would you want to eat the plastic bag? Of course not. You need to filter, or remove, the chlorine before drinking the water. A carbon filter will remove gaseous chemicals and impurities such as chlorine, but it will not remove essential minerals. These type filters are widely available on the retail market.

OXYGEN

There is a great deal of controversy surrounding this subject. Again, keep things simple. Oxygen is extremely healing in all aspects. No, it is not a cure for cancer. There is not a cure for cancer either in the conventional world or the alternative world. Oxygen can be used safely and with no side effects, so why not incorporate some form of oxygen therapy?

There are several forms of oxygen therapies out there which include hyperbaric therapy, ozonizing, and hydrogen peroxide. Hyperbaric therapy is done in a pressurized chamber. It uses 100% oxygen under pressure. This increased oxygen means that the blood is carrying more oxygen to the cells, which leads to substantial cell repair. Ozone therapy is effective because rather than O2 it has an extra oxygen molecule, O3, which also gives the blood cells more oxygen. A high amount of oxygen kills viruses and disease and facilitates immune function. Hydrogen peroxide therapy is yet another form of oxygen supply to the blood. This therapy is done intravenously by drawing the patients' blood, mixing it with hydrogen peroxide, and injecting it back into the patient. These are non-harmful ways to support the body in healing.

Oxygen is the breath of life. When the body is sick it needs more of everything from nutrition to water to oxygen. We take these things for granted, but they are readily available in safe, nontoxic therapies. Look into how you can supply your body with life-sustaining oxygen.

TOXINS IN THE ENVIRONMENT

We are exposed to a multitude of toxins in our environment from the air we breathe to the phones we use. Our bodies are under attack every day. Please do not freak out over this, just become aware of your surroundings and make minor changes. Also, remember that your skin is the largest organ of the body. It is alive and it absorbs everything you touch, so wear gloves. That is easy. Look at the ingredients of the lotions and soaps you put on your body. If you cannot eat it, then you should not use it. There are some great natural brands that do not contain so many chemicals and toxins.

EMF—ELECTRO MAGNETIC FIELDS

✌ I want to talk about EMF because my husband was exposed to high levels on the carrier and in the cockpit. This is a serious toxin that is not seen or felt. We are exposed to it on a daily basis with our cell phones, electric blankets, alarm clocks, computers, TV's, and more. We think nothing of sitting in front of a computer all day and we wonder why we are so fatigued at the end of the day. Our bodies are fighting the disruption of energy caused by EMF.

Electricity is an inseparable part of our modern day society. This means EMF will continue to be all around us. Aside from making our lives easier, electricity is also making our lives shorter. EMF from power lines, home wiring, airport and military radar, substations, transformers, computers and appliances, cause brain tumors, leukemia, birth defects, miscarriages, chronic fatigue, headaches, cataracts, heart problems, stress, nausea, chest pain, forgetfulness, cancer, and many other health problems.

Numerous studies have produced contradictory results, yet some experts are convinced that the threat is real. By 1990, over one hundred studies had been conducted worldwide. Of these, at least two dozen indicated a link between EMF and serious health problems. This is not something to be ignored just because we cannot see or feel it. More studies are under way. The large cell phone companies, the military, and electric companies do not want this information to reach consumers, so the process is slow. Please make sure you use an ear bud or blue tooth for your cell phone. Do not use an electric blanket and put your alarm clock at least four feet away from your head. Do not stand next to a microwave while it is running. Actually, leave the room. There are devices out there to help diffuse EMF from computers and power boxes. Become aware of your surroundings and make adjustments in your home.

Here's the Deal: Cancer Cells Are Different from Healthy Cells

✓ Otto Warburg discovered that cancer cells are anaerobic (without oxygen) and healthy cells are aerobic (with oxygen).

✓ We are responsible for creating the environment in which cancer thrives.

✓ Cancer cells have a lack of nutrition, oxygen, and hydration.

Here's the Deal:
There Is an Environment in which Cancer Lives!

✓ Oxidative stress damages cells on a daily basis so you need antioxidants to neutralize this effect.

✓ Nutritionally, Americans are the most overfed yet malnourished people on the planet.

✓ Nutrient-dense foods are packed full of life-sustaining nutrition and should be part of your everyday intake of food.

✓ Sugar feeds cancer. Read your labels. Four grams of sugar = 1 teaspoon of sugar.

✓ Food enzymes are involved in every process in the body and are only found in live raw foods.

✓ Processed foods are denatured and lacking in nutrient value. They do more harm than good.

✓ Partially hydrogenated oil (trans fat) is

harmful to the body. It is a preservative to keep food on the shelves, NOT to keep you healthy.

✓ Inflammation helps cancer grow. Increase your omega 3 (fish, flax, nuts) and decrease omega 6 (animal fat) to help decrease inflammation.

✓ Cancer loves an acidic environment. This is created by lack of water, oxygen, nutrition, and sleep.

✓ Water is essential to good health. A gallon a day is not too much.

✓ Oxygen is the breath of life and leads to healing and cell repair. There are multiple methods to increase your oxygen: Hyperbaric, ozonating, and hydrogen peroxide.

✓ Toxins in the environment bombard our bodies every day. Though unseen and unfelt, EMF disrupt the cellular function of our bodies.

Here's the Deal: Control your Environment

✓ You really can control the environment in which cancer lives.

✓ Choices you make really do make a difference: what you eat, where you live, how you live, and peace of mind.

✓ You are not a victim of the disease. Your immune system is impaired so do what you can to rebuild it.

✓ Knowledge is the key, so don't dismiss things just because you have never been told about them. Read food labels, ask how supplements work, and understand on a cellular level what is happening and what you want to achieve.

Chapter
SEVEN

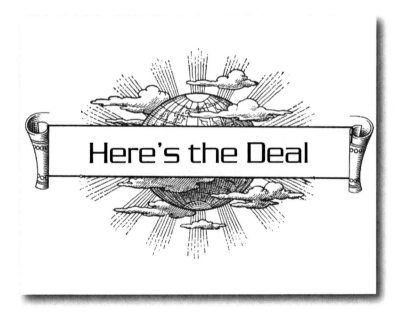

Here's the Deal

THE WHOLE BODY

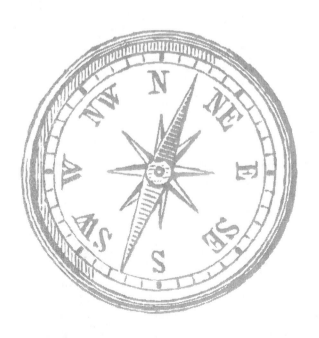

DETOXIFICATION

✍ One of the easiest ways to improve your quality of life is detoxification. Detoxifying the body cleans out toxins that have built up over the years. This buildup weakens the ability of cells to function correctly which ultimately weakens the immune system.

Detoxification means reducing, removing, neutralizing, eliminating, and avoiding toxins. Toxins are substances that are harmful to the body. They interfere with chemical reactions, metabolism, nerve transmission, and cellular structure.

A detoxification program assists the body in removing unwanted or poisonous materials created by the process of normal living. All toxic substances cannot be readily dumped out of the body. They must stand in line and wait their turn to exit through limited avenues. Some damage from toxic substances occurs while they are waiting for their turn to be eliminated.

The liver is one of the most important organs for building up and tearing down chemicals created by the body. There are certain nutrients the liver requires in large amounts to facilitate this function. We need to consider assisting the liver to cleanse itself.

The bowel is the second major detoxification organ. Not only can bacteria, fungi, parasites, and viruses proliferate in the bowel, but, through the leaky gut walls, some of them can gain entrance to the interior of the body to create havoc. That is why constipation is so detrimental to health.

The blood is another major detoxification element, but only as long as it is moving adequately through the body. Oxygen is the key to maintaining good blood flow as well as reducing blood sludge (the thickening of the blood due to dehydration and lack of oxygen). Oxygen can be considered the most effective and efficient detoxifying ingredient known to man.

The kidneys, as long as they are not overloaded and are working properly, are also major detoxifying organs. Perhaps the most important function of the kidneys is to assist in the removal of excess positively-charged minerals from the body. To accomplish filtration and mineral removal adequately, the kidneys must have a good blood supply and there must be enough water in the system. The kidneys require more water than most people consume. So increasing your water to a minimum of eight glasses per day can significantly assist your kidneys to function properly.

To sum it up, toxemia is a potential problem for most of us. It will sap energy and reduce resistance to other problems that might afflict us. Our organs are strained and do not function optimally when we are fighting disease. It is up to us to help our bodies function correctly. Incorporating therapies such as colon hydrotherapy, coffee enemas, and pro-biotic enzyme supplements will help organs and boost immunity. Detox programs led by professionals such as chiropractors, naturopaths, therapists, and physicians are safe and effective in helping jump-start your body.

LYMPHATIC DRAINAGE

Lymphatic drainage is a specialized, manual technique designed to activate and cleanse the human fluid system. Because the lymphatic system itself is responsible for optimum functioning of the water circulation and immune system, it is a key to maximizing your ability to rejuvenate and to establish resistance to stress and disease. This work is facilitated by medical professionals including physical therapists, occupational therapists, nurses, and massage therapists who are specially trained in this technique.

Your lymphatic system - the immune system - is an independently-functioning system in the body. It has its own network of capillaries, channels, and nodes. Its job is to help the body get rid of anything and everything it doesn't use on a cellular level. It takes care of the larger proteins that cannot enter the blood capillaries. It also allows unrecognized particles and molecules to be absorbed into the lymph capillaries. And guess what? It destroys viruses, bacteria, and diseases that are in the body. Without this vital system, we would die!

The way it works is actually very simple. The lymph capillaries are not like blood capillaries. A blood capillary is similar to a straw that has an opening at each end and is solid in the middle. A lymph capillary has overlapping filaments much like fish gills. These filaments are attached to the derma of the skin. Any kind of movement helps open these filaments and allows larger particles and fluid to enter.

You have Lymph nodes all over your body. However, there are several major "dumping stations" or node areas. These are on the neck, under the arms, and at the crease of the legs. The function of the nodes is to destroy foreign matter or toxins. If these nodes are full (too much for the body to handle) there is a "traffic jam" and toxins cannot exit the body. This will make you very sick.

The same is true if you have an injury or surgery. The extra inflammation or fluid is absorbed into the lymphatic system, which takes care of swelling. Swelling is your body's natural protection when it is traumatized. In addition, when you've had surgery, you're given pain medications, anesthesia, etc. This causes additional toxins in the body, which inundates the lymph system. This, coupled with additional swelling, totally overloads the lymph nodes.

There really is no medication for the lymph system itself, so manual therapy is the best way to help the system, assisting the body to "dump" toxins and heal faster. If you are suffering from a chronic illness or recovering from surgery, lymph drainage therapy is critical in your recovery. Manually moving fluids and assisting the nodes to dump and refill, greatly improves the capacity of the lymph and helps lessen pain.

Tommy always felt so much better after manual lymph drainage. It helped his body eliminate toxins giving him more energy and making him feel less sluggish. This therapy was effective in stimulating the immune function so it could fight the cancer while cleaning up the toxic medications and other cellular debris due to the disease. It lowered inflammation and the overall stress level on his body. In Tommy's case, this was a very effective therapy.

The next best thing to help improve lymph function and actually prevent sickness is limiting exposure to toxic foods. If you put a denatured substance into your body, let's say processed food, your body cannot recognize it. These toxins are then sent to the lymph because they're unusable by the cells. The lymph is forced to divert from fighting disease to working on the toxins you added. In other words, by eating that Twinkie, you've just side-tracked the lymph from doing its major job of fighting viruses and disease to being a garbage disposal for the empty food you ate. Don't assume that cookies and chips just turn into fat. They're actually harmful and lower your immune function. Fresh fruits, vegetables, and plenty of water are what every human body desperately needs. They help the lymph system because the body recognizes them as fuel and because there's very little debris for the lymph to handle. Instead, the nodes can work on keeping you well.

MASSAGE THERAPY

Massage Therapy is your key to getting a handle on total well-being. Massage treats the whole body from the inside out. It brings blood and oxygen to the tissues and makes you aware of aches and pains so you can address and prevent problems. It also trains you to let go and relax. This is a key element to getting along in this society. Stress is all around us and having the ability to recognize tension (the way we sit, the way we breathe, the gripping of the shoulders and neck) and knowing how to let it go will increase whole-body health. With massage therapy, your adrenal glands will calm down (fight or flight mode), your blood pressure will lower, your oxygen flow will increase by taking deep breaths, you will be able to digest food properly (reflux, IBS, colitis), and more. By having regular massage therapy, you will get to know your body and learn techniques from your massage therapist to correct tension, relieve pain, stretch and isolate muscles, and live healthier.

As you can see from the table on page 132, there is a vast difference between spa massage, therapeutic massage, and oncology massage. All have an important role to play, but not all are suitable to everyone. I have heard over and over that people give their girlfriends a spa package after their chemo treatments to "give them a day off." This is one of the last things you want to do for someone with a compromised immune system who is battling a disease! Each type of massage requires specific training. If a breast cancer survivor goes to a spa it is most likely the therapist has not been trained in lymph node drainage, port sites, chemo-induced fragility of the skin, neuropathy, radiation burns, etc. A deep tissue message or even a Swedish massage could make this individual extremely sick due to the improper use of pressure and overstimulation of an impaired immune system. Spa Massage is basically for well individuals. It is for those experiencing stress on a day-to-day basis, not for those encountering life-threatening disease.

Therapeutic massage is very different as well. The training a therapist receives in order to be effective in this area is focused on problem-solving. This type of massage is most common for sports and post-surgery. The tissues are worked in a much more aggressive manner in order to restore full range of motion to a joint or other area. Scars are addressed by breaking up the adhesions to underlying areas developed by the scar tissues. Muscles that are gripped and guarded due to protecting an injury or surgery are released with deep neuromuscular techniques. Blood and oxygen are brought to restricted areas with specific cross-friction techniques. As you can see, therapeutic massage is very different from spa massage. Yes, pain is eventually relieved with therapeutic massage, but the process is far from relaxing!

Oncology massage takes a whole new approach to the healing process. It is not focused on problem-solving. Instead, it is focused on accepting the individual just where they are in the healing process. Cancer treatments are invasive and extremely stressful. The anxiety levels of cancer patients are at an all-time high. Not only are they faced with the "diagnosis" they've received, but now they are faced with very toxic, life-threatening treatments. Individuals going through all this also tend to disconnect from themselves. It is difficult to accept that the cancer is a part of them. They can either talk about "the cancer" or about themselves, but not together. Gentle touch is very effective in bringing down the anxiety and renewing the mind-body connection. Studies have shown a 60% reduction in treatment side effects with just twenty minutes of gentle touch. The pressure is very light and the strokes are long and slow. There are specific techniques to relieve pain that can be very nurturing and helpful to the individual. This therapy allows the client to "let go" and breathe. When anxiety is lowered, the body kicks into gear. Digestion improves, immune function is boosted, blood flow is increased, insomnia is reduced, and healing begins - all with the trained hands of an oncology massage therapist.

As I mentioned earlier, not all massage is the same. Incorporate one that fits your needs and experience a greater quality of life.

HERE'S THE DEAL ABOUT CANCER

	Spa Massage	Therapeutic Massage	Oncology Massage
Intent	Relaxation	Problem Solving	Acceptance
	Stress Release	Relieve Pain	Comfort
	Reward/Pamper	Improve ROM	Reduce Anxiety
	Improve Skin Appearance	Reduce Inflammation	Assist Immune Function
	Feel Good	Reduce Scaring	Reduce Pain
			Mind/Body Connection
Technique	Swedish/Deep Tissue	Scar Therapy	Light Touch
	Hot Stones	Lymph Drainage	Gentle Muscle Release
	Aromatherapy	Neuromuscular	Manual Lymph Drainage
	Body Wraps	Trigger Points	Remain Clothed
	Manicure/Pedicure	Cross Friction	Focus: Hands/Feet/Head
	Facials	Myofacial Release	
		Sports Massage	
Result	Deep Relaxation	Reduced Pain	Reduced Anxiety
	Improved Skin Appearance	Faster Healing	Improved Immune Function
	Reduced Stress	Improved ROM	Increased Blood Flow
	Improved Circulation	Increased Pliability of Tissues (soft and elastic)	Improved Digestion
	Increased Oxygen and Blood Flow	Reduced Swelling	Improved Sleep
	Body Awareness	Reduced Scarring	Self-Empowerment
		Relieved Muscle Tension	Mind/Body Connection

QUALITY OF LIFE

～ You will begin to notice a significant increase in the quality of your life once you begin to feel better. Doctors were not telling us this information and, for a while, I thought I was bucking the system. I mean, who in the heck was I to go up against brain surgeons and brain doctors? I was just a concerned, loving housewife.

But, as we started to change our diet and supplements, we saw changes in Tommy (no symptoms) and on his brain scan (no growth). The tumor stopped growing so we knew the alternative treatments were working. If you think of it logically, healing comes from how God made our bodies. It just makes sense to add the whole body piece to the puzzle. Being proactive and taking care of our bodies, added to the puzzle of wellness, gives the cells what they need to do their job - fight the cancer. Some institutions and hospitals are actually combining nutrition with the treatment of cancer and realizing the connection between nutrition and disease.

I discovered that the medical community is limited in knowledge of whole-body wellness. Studies concerning the impact of manual touch therapies on the healing process are just now coming out. We are a society of treating symptoms and giving medications. There is nothing wrong with that except that sometimes it takes more of a hands-on approach to heal the body. When you are faced with a terminal disease such as cancer, a whole-body approach is necessary. You are looking at long-term treatment, not just a few doctor visits. You are also looking at death as the final outcome if aggressive procedures are not done. Chemical regimens are exhausting, taxing, and devastating. Incorporating manual therapies and things you can do at home brings about a more nurturing aspect of healing and a whole body empowerment.

There is no magic bullet out there. Healing requires a combination of treatments to optimize results. The idea is to help your body fight the disease. In order to do this you have to build up the immune system. To build the immune system the body has to recognize and utilize the nutrients you put into it. For long-term results, you cannot "trick" the body with drugs. You have to boost it with nutrients.

Educate yourself little bits at the time on foods and toxins and their relationships to disease. Your body is working hard to fight the cancer. Read food labels along with the ingredients section. Carefully and specifically look for bleached, enriched flour, high fructose corn syrup, and partially hydrogenated oils. When you have a sickness, eliminating toxins from your food is an absolute must. The idea is to get your body into a state where it can heal itself and stop the growth of the tumor or whatever is contributing to your illness. If you create a strong immune system and an environment where the tumor or illness cannot grow, you have a better long-term chance of fighting the disease.

Start eliminating the bad and incorporating the good. You will experience a greater quality of life. When you feel better and start contributing to your long-term healing, you will be empowered and have a say in the way your life will be lived.

Here's the Deal: What Do You Want the Therapy to Do?

✓   Don't do a therapy just because it is "supposed" to help. Ask yourself what it is supposed TO DO to help your body.

✓   Incorporating therapies assists the body to

heal. It is not a magic bullet.

✓ Know the end result you are trying to achieve to improve the quality of life.

✓ Ask yourself if the therapy or supplement is bringing down inflammation, blocking receptors, feeding the tumor, starving the tumor, balancing acidity, hydrating to help detoxification, or hydrating to absorb nutrients. Get the picture?

Here's the Deal: Stick to a Plan; then Re-evaluate

✓ Give yourself a month to determine if a therapy is working.

✓ Be intentional about the incorporation of the therapy or change you have made. (If you say you are going to increase your water intake, drink a gallon of water a day, not just a few glasses.)

✓ You may experience changes (for example: bloating, increased urination, lack of sleep). This is not necessarily a "bad" thing; it is just a change, so try to work through it.

✓ Re-evaluate your quality of life monthly. If something is not working or if there is an overlapping of therapies, make necessary changes and continue with a plan. If you do not have a plan of action, incorporating changes to help your body heal will be more difficult to achieve and less positive results will be accomplished.

Here's the Deal: Cleanse the Body

✓ Detoxification means reducing, removing, neutralizing, eliminating, and avoiding toxins.

✓ Due to the effects of disease on the body, our organs do not function properly. We have to help them by incorporating detoxification therapies.

Here's the Deal: The Lymph System is our Immune System

✓ The Lymph system is made up of its own nodes, capillaries, and channels that function independently.

✓ When you are sick, the nodes become overloaded and toxins build up in the body.

✓ Lymph Drainage Therapy will assist the lymph system in taking on and dumping more unwanted toxins from the body which, in turn, will help you feel better and fight your sickness more effectively.

✓ Lymph Therapy is an essential component in the fight against cancer.

Here's the Deal: Massage Therapy = Total Wellbeing

✓ There are differences between spa massage, therapeutic massage, and oncology massage.

✓ Therapeutic massage is focused on problem solving.

✓ Oncology massage is focused on accepting the individual just where they are in the healing process. It could involve lymph drainage, Healing Touch, and light massage.

✓ Spa massage focuses on well individuals experiencing stress on a day-to-day basis.

Chapter
EIGHT

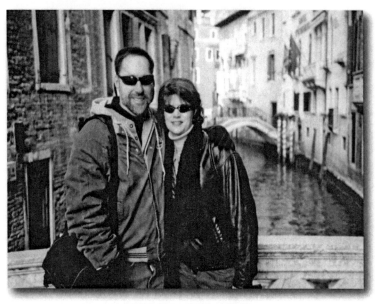

Venice Italy, October 2005

INTEGRATE
THERAPIES

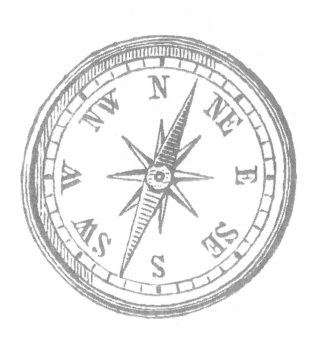

❦ We decided to hold off on the chemo a little longer. The Protocel, along with the supplements and diet, seemed to be working. The last few MRIs showed a lot of highlight in the pons, speech, and frontal lobe. However, the PET scans showed only active tumor in the pons. This confirmed that it wasn't tumor growth. Also, Tom had very few symptoms. His speech was messed up a little and he had to concentrate on some words, but he was still fluent. He felt great, worked full-time, and exercised. The doctors were even puzzled as to why he wasn't experiencing more symptoms. We'd tried to explain to them about our therapies but they didn't want to hear about it. Our neuro-oncologists were an important part of our treatment team. We didn't argue with them, but always kept them informed of what we were doing. They weren't very supportive of our ideas. However, they were not discouraging.

The doctors said Tom was a miracle. I tended to stay very guarded and just lived month to month. He was so awesome about all of it. I loved him so much!

Keeping up a daily regimen of supplements wasn't easy. We had to make some adjustments. We ended up getting little plastic pill bottles from the pharmacy and labeling them - morning, breakfast, midmorning, lunch, mid-afternoon, dinner, and bedtime. That helped a lot. Tommy also set his alarm on his watch so he'd remember to take them.

JANUARY 2005

༄ We'd managed to stay off chemo for 10 months. Tommy was doing great. His speech had been a little worse and he was having balance issues. I cringed when he told me, but at the same time, I wanted to know. He had been having some headaches and was interested in getting back on the steroid. I was concerned, so I called our nutritionist and supplement advisor and a distributor of the Protocel to see what it could be. I thought it was swelling, but from what? The general consensus was it probably indicated fluid buildup from the tumor cells dying. Ordinarily, the body would re-absorb that fluid, but for some reason, Tommy was holding on to it. He was taking four different natural supplements for inflammation. We knew he might have to start a stronger prescription anti-inflammatory plus a steroid.

FEBRUARY 2005

༄ Things were about the same. Tommy started the steroid at a low dose. He still took his supplements and watched what he ate. The latest symptoms were talking gibberish, 30-minute spans of not understanding people, pressure in his head, and balance issues. We felt this was the dying off of cancer cells and his being unable to get rid of the debris or mucus caused by that. He drank a lot of water and tried to get a lot of rest. We hoped this would help the symptoms improve.

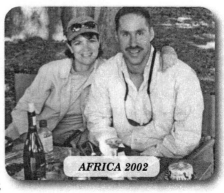

AFRICA 2002

Tom had good days and bad days with his speech. He took the steroid and that helped with the balance issues. He drank more water and actually got rid of some of the mucus through his scalp. It looked like a bad case of dandruff. It was also on his face. He said that when he urinated, it bubbled. We felt these things indicated more elimination of dead cancer cells.

Just think, it had been a year since Tommy's last chemo treatment. We had come so far in that year. I truly believed in whole food nutrition. I believed in getting your body to work for you instead of against you. I also believed that all supplements are not for everyone. It depends on the makeup of each person's body and what they are trying to accomplish.

MARCH 2005

≈ Tommy had another MRI and it basically said he was still lit up, but no change. We got a call from the doctors and they weren't happy with what they were seeing. I still believed the MRI showed swelling with broken-up tumor and mucus making it look like a large mass. I believed this because the highlights on the MRI were a dull gray, not a bright, solid mass. Also, I knew Tommy would have more symptoms and be more disabled if all those areas were being taken over by the tumor. The conventional doctors weren't familiar with that type of breakup. They were only accustomed to the whole tumor shrinking and interpreting the scans the way they had been taught.

Tommy's quality of life was great! He was fully functional. Our approach was still working. I hated the uncertainty about the MRI and wanted him to

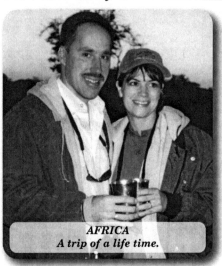

AFRICA
A trip of a life time.

get a PET scan before we decided on any more chemo. That was extremely difficult. I didn't want to hurt him. I wished something would happen so we would know for sure. I hated that feeling of "here we go again."

Tommy and I decided to go ahead and make an appointment with the oncologist to hear what he had to say. We also scheduled a PET scan so we would have all of the information in front of us. The doctors wanted to do a biopsy to see if the cancer had mutated into a more aggressive tumor.

It was interesting to see how the conventional world and alternative world couldn't work together. It was truly up to the individual to integrate the two. We had just found out that our insurance company case manager who was handling Tommy's case was dropped without our knowledge. I was livid! Why would they drop the case in the middle of treatment? Well, I soon realized that Tommy wasn't in the middle of "their" treatment. The insurance company said that, because Tommy had

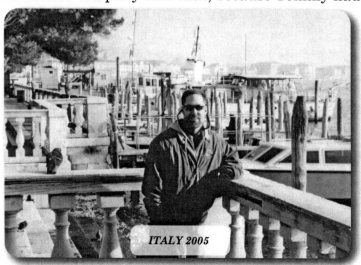

ITALY 2005

not received chemo for a year, he was no longer considered eligible for a case manager. Needless to say, I got another case manager assigned, but that had been an eye-opening experience of the measures conventional medicine use compared to the measures of true health and wellness.

I had been praying for God to intervene if this was not the way we should go. Well, he did just that. The hospital couldn't perform the biopsy on the day we had scheduled, so there was no need for us to go. Also, the PET scan results came back and they were about the same with warm spots in the speech area. The doctors were baffled with these reports and determined the scans were inconclusive. I was excited! God had answered our prayers! Why start a toxic treatment that would break down the immunity and have horrible side effects when the nontoxic regimen was holding things at bay and giving Tommy a good quality of life?

APRIL 2005

✎ Time was flying by. I couldn't believe it had been so long since we had been in Mexico. The whole family was feeling great with our new lifestyle. The kids were off their allergy medications. I was off my IBS medication. Tommy was feeling great and off the chemo. We had settled into a workable routine to keep everything going.

Food took up a large chunk of my day, but I knew it made all the difference in the world. I actually enjoyed finding new foods and recipes. It was amazing how flavorful the spices and herbs were compared with the bland, fatty foods we had eaten previously. I seasoned our foods with olive oils and spices instead of fat and salt. We used honey and stevia instead of refined sugar. I made my own bread from fresh wheat. I actually ground the wheat and made the flour. The glycemic index of freshly ground wheat is much lower. The family had adjusted and loved the new menu.

Tommy had not detoxed for some time so we started incorporating more detoxification treatments into our routine. We were seeing a naturopathic doctor to help with this process. Also, to stimulate the liver to dump more efficiently, we decided to do coffee enemas. At first, they sounded extreme. However, after educating ourselves, we discovered they were actually very noninvasive and the benefits were huge.

MAY 2005

Another month passed and we still had not been to our oncologist. Tommy was doing great! He was off the steroid completely! We were still seeing the naturopath and incorporating detoxification into our routine. Tommy's symptoms were better. His speech was about 80/20 and he had some balance issues when playing golf. Hmmm, tough life!

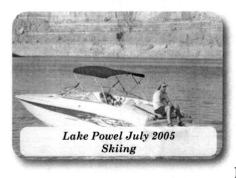

Lake Powel July 2005
Skiing

Now that I'd learned so much about nutrition and how the body worked, I talked about it all the time. I just wanted to tell as many people as I could that they could actually prevent cancer by making a few lifestyle changes. Increasing water intake could lower cancer risk by up to 60%. Overcooking vegetables removes the nutrient value of raw or lightly steamed vegetables. Why not make some adjustments and get the most out of your food?

I have to vent a little here. The downside of my enthusiasm was anger and lack of patience. I found myself getting short with people when they made excuses and wouldn't listen to my advice. I mean, I was living the wake-up call and finding out that just changing a few things could have prevented this from happening, and a lot of people just didn't want to hear it. They had no interest in making any changes. I guess they thought it was hard enough getting through life.

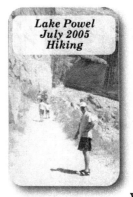

Lake Powel July 2005 Hiking

Another thing I was angry about was the fact that our medical system teaches treatment, not prevention. You only go to the doctor when you're sick. In fact, doctors don't want to see you unless you're sick because they don't practice preventative medicine. It's always wait and see. Wait and see what? That the cancer has grown? That the IBS is worse? That the infections have spread? Why not prevent these things from happening by incorporating healthy eating?

Needless to say, my passion came across as, "You're wrong," instead of, "Wow, did you know . . .?" So, I tended to offend or scare people. That made me sad and was totally not my intent. I often prayed for patience.

SEPTEMBER 2005

It had been several months and Tommy was feeling some new symptoms. He was experiencing pressure in his head when he bent over and he had more balance issues. The doctor said the tumors looked worse and were growing down the brain stem. We decided to set up an appointment to have a PET scan and figure out a plan. The doctors wanted to do a different trial than they had suggested a year before. I asked why and they said that the first one wasn't as effective as this new one. I was so glad we waited. I'd done my homework on the new one before we went to the appointment.

I got on the computer and did my research. The more I read about chemo the more I didn't want Tommy to do it. On the other hand, maybe the chemo would get us on top of this thing for the short term and we could maintain the growth with

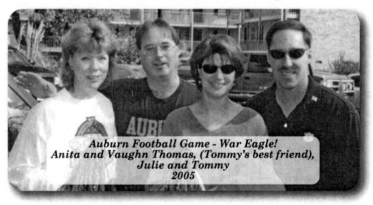

Auburn Football Game - War Eagle!
Anita and Vaughn Thomas, (Tommy's best friend),
Julie and Tommy
2005

alternative methods. It was interesting that I was actually starting to understand the medical jargon and knew how to read trials and protocols. Who would have ever guessed a finance major could learn all of that?

JANUARY 2006

✎   The past three months had been a roller coaster to say the least. The following bullet points sum it up:

- We revamped the supplement schedule and incorporated more anti-inflammatory products hoping that they would relieve the pressure in the brain.

- We followed an alkalizing diet for six weeks which limited the foods we could eat and made Tommy lose 10 pounds. An alkalizing diet is good, but it just didn't work for our family. We tried alkalizing drops in the water instead.

- Tommy's symptoms started getting worse: balance, speech, fatigue, and his ability to fill in the gap while talking (everything had to be explained).

- Tommy went back on chemo. We went to the neuro-oncologist and decided to start the trial chemo in order to shock the tumors and get on top of the growth.

- Tommy had a bad reaction to the chemo. His brain swelled and all aspects of functioning were impaired: he couldn't talk (speech), walk (balance), eat (got sick due to imbalance, not the drugs), reason (didn't know what was going on), just to name a few.

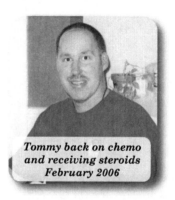

Tommy back on chemo and receiving steroids February 2006

- We took Tom to an immune clinic in Atlanta to be extremely aggressive in building his immunity to help him handle the chemo treatments. He was put on an IV drip very similar to what he experienced in Mexico. They also incorporated other therapies to help balance his body.

- After a few weeks of immune therapies you couldn't even tell he had been on chemo therapy. They boosted his body so it could handle the toxins from the chemo and allowed his body to balance itself. He could function normally.

- We went to the immune clinic every day. It took the whole day to receive the therapies. He had all of his functions back and was able to handle the second round of chemotherapy much better.

- Witnessing the drastic changes in Tommy really confirmed the importance of combining therapies. It was the key in experiencing greater quality of life while going through cancer treatment.

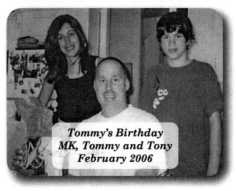

Tommy's Birthday
MK, Tommy and Tony
February 2006

- After six weeks, the scans showed fewer enhancements. I knew the combination of immune therapies, diet, and chemo, were the factors in getting rid of the tumors. It wasn't just the chemo alone. Also, Tommy was feeling and doing much better with his immunity boosted. Others in his position who weren't doing immune therapies were very, very, sick.

- Tommy stopped working and was on short-term disability until the end of the year. He would go on long-term disability if needed. He had to take time off work to go full-time to the immune clinic. The clinic made such a difference in his quality of life it was well worth going every day.

• Tommy's initiative improved and he was making to-do lists. Every now and then he would get tired, but not sick. His bowels were loud and gassy but basically okay. Considering he was on chemotherapy, you would think they would be much worse. I knew the immune therapy was making the difference.

• We were on the right track. So far, so good. But we were not out of the woods yet!

❧ I want to talk about the immune clinic for just a bit. We went to the Immune Recovery Foundation in Georgia. It was wonderful that they were right here in Atlanta. This is a wonderful healing environment. It's the ultimate at combining conventional and alternative methods under one roof. They look at immediate issues and address them with medications yet still look at the whole body and address quality of life issues with alternative methods. The dosage of medication is minimal because they use high doses of vitamin C to carry the medications where they need to go. The people there are wonderful. It was like our extended family. The atmosphere was much like Mexico. They use lots of different therapies but on a laid-back schedule. Each day you don't know which therapies you'll be receiving. There are no worries, though, you just rest in big, comfortable recliners and the staff comes to you and gets you going.

One of the most effective therapies Tommy received was lymphatic drainage. We learned that the lymph system is your immune system. It gathers toxins and substances not used by the body and gets rid of them. When manual lymph therapy is done, it helps the immunity by getting more toxins to the lymph nodes to be dumped so even more can be removed from the system. Tommy actually felt better physically after this therapy. He looked forward to his lymph drainage sessions.

I still don't understand why insurance companies don't cover those therapies while people are on heavy drugs like chemo. I don't understand why immune drips aren't given while chemo is given. Doctors know that chemo lowers the immunity, so why can't they give nutrients to help boost it? I've asked the medical staff about this while in IV rooms. They always say they're not specialized in that area. They only treat the cancer. If we wanted to boost the immunity, we would have to take some sort of other drug or speak to a nutritionist. This was just further verification that the worlds of conventional medicine and alternative methods don't blend.

APRIL 2006

⚮   Tommy received two more rounds of chemo while receiving the immune therapies. His personality started to change. He became more childlike and had extreme mood changes. When we spoke to the doctors about it, they said it sounded like he was becoming bipolar due to the chemo. They wanted to prescribe a very strong bipolar medication to help.

Mary and I were not comfortable with this.

*   We knew the medications were causing this change in behavior, not the tumors.

*   We knew that Tommy's quality of life was the most important thing and that the behavior issue was taking away from that.

*   We were not impressed by survival rate statistics with chemo.

*   We knew the drug Tom was taking with this chemo, which made it very effective against brain cancer, was also restricting blood flow to his brain.

*   We decided to discontinue the chemo but continue with the immune clinic. We felt the

chemo's job was done. The tumors had shrunk and Tommy was better.

If not for the research and knowledge we had gained over the past two years, we wouldn't have been comfortable taking Tommy off the chemo. The doctors weren't happy with our decision, but we were looking after his quality of life, not just getting rid of the tumors.

JUNE 2006

After six months with the immune clinic, Tommy went back to work part-time. Because of all the swelling and therapies, his ability to sort out numbers was an issue. His boss was great and gave him small tasks to work on. It was important for Tommy to get back into the saddle and work. We were still on short-term disability so he could only work part-time. This actually worked out well because he felt a bit run down by the end of the day.

SEPTEMBER 2006

Tommy was doing so much better being off the chemotherapy protocol. We had made plans to go to Hawaii for our 20th wedding anniversary. Tom's parents wanted to give us the trip to celebrate. We had never been to Hawaii and couldn't wait to get away.

Hawaii was wonderful. We stayed on the Island of Kauai in a time share condo on the beach. To my surprise, Tommy did great on the flight. I was worried about the pressure on the brain with such a long flight. We took advantage of every activity. We took a zodiac around the coastline of the island, rode four-wheelers in the forests, played in the waterfalls, toured the

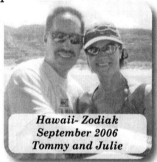

Hawaii- Zodiak
September 2006
Tommy and Julie

pineapple and coffee farms, went to a luau, took helicopter rides, hiked, and just enjoyed relaxing with each other. Does that sound like someone with a brain tumor?

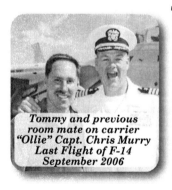

Tommy and previous
room mate on carrier
"Ollie" Capt. Chris Murry
Last Flight of F-14
September 2006

Tommy got to reunite with his flying buddies and witness the last flight of the F-14. It was a wonderful reunion of his comrades and friends that had been such an important part of our lives. The ceremony was held at NAS Oceana in Virginia Beach, VA. Tommy

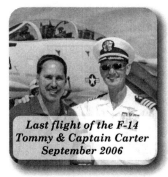

Last flight of the F-14
Tommy & Captain Carter
September 2006

and I loved being with our Navy Family and remembering such great times we spent together. Everyone seemed genuinely happy to see him. I could see the light in Tommy's eyes as he went down memory lane with his comrades. It totally warmed my heart. He has sacrificed so much with this disease, yet he has never asked "why me?" No one knew the tumors were still active, which again showed another level of quality of life Tommy experienced. He did not want to appear "sick" to his buddies and was able to be his old self for one whole weekend! We were so totally blessed to experience this event and bring closure to his flying career. He was truly amazing!

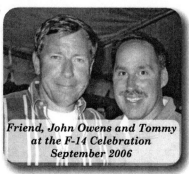

Friend, John Owens and Tommy
at the F-14 Celebration
September 2006

OCTOBER 2006

✎ I started massage school so that I could learn lymph drainage. I wanted to be able to do that for Tommy on a regular basis because it made such a difference for him. I found a school near my house that had fantastic hours and the right accreditations. It was a good outlet for me as I wanted to learn more about the body.

Tom had been off chemo for a while and we had stopped the immune therapies. His behavior had improved and things were going well. He still worked part-time and we talked to his boss about possibly going full-time. We had a strict supplement routine and were keeping to the diet. The whole food eating was just a way of life for us now. Bad foods seemed to upset our stomachs and we really didn't even have a desire for them. The only thing Tommy seemed to crave was sugar. Remember what I said earlier? Cancer feeds on sugar!

Here's the Deal: Steps to Integrate Treatments

Okay, you're open to integrating your treatment and understanding the importance of detox and nutrition. Where do you begin?

✓ Just because your cancer isn't responding doesn't mean the fight is over.

✓ Educate yourself on your disease.

✓ Use resources at the library and online.

✓ Ask questions.

✓ Educate yourself on alternative therapies.

✓ Put together your own team to address your specific situation.

✓ Weed out your pantry.

✓ Rework your normal day to find time to exercise and prepare meals.

✓ Slow down your lifestyle.

✓ Limit stress.

✓ Get adequate rest.

✓ Drink filtered water and lots of it.

✓ Start building your knowledge base.

✓ Rework your budget so that you'll have funds

to pursue therapies which are not covered by insurance.

Here's the Deal:
Kick Your Body into Action

✓ You have to detoxify the body because sludge and trash cause disease and interfere with immune function.

✓ The body will kick into action when it's given what it needs to function correctly.

✓ Giving your body the nutrients it needs is better medicine than any pharmaceuticals.

Here's the Deal:
Work WITH, Not AGAINST your Doctors

✓ Get regular scans to determine cancer growth.

✓ Tell the doctors what you're doing. I guarantee you that if they were in your shoes, they would do the same thing.

✓ Don't look for medical doctors to advise you on diet and supplements. This is out of their scope of practice and they aren't allowed to do so.

✓ Incorporate a naturopathic doctor, nutritionist, or chiropractor that specializes in supplementation to help with alternative therapies.

✓ Do your research on the therapies you're incorporating.

Here's the Deal:
Combine the Two Therapies

✓ Create an environment where cancer cannot live (less acidity, less inflammation, less sugar for energy, less processed food, and more fruits and vegetables to help immune function, less stress to reduce free radical activity, and less negative living to appreciate and enjoy how precious life is).

✓ Sometimes natural, less-toxic means of treatment aren't aggressive enough, so traditional medicines are necessary to get the disease under control.

✓ Combining traditional and alternative methods will enhance the effects of the chemo and balance the body so it can handle the toxins.

✓ Chemotherapy kills cells and alternative methods support and bring life to cells. It just makes sense to incorporate both treatments.

✓ There is no magic bullet. It takes a combination of therapies to slow growth of a disease.

Here's the Deal:
The Missing Link

✓ When you're first diagnosed with cancer, you're only given three options: surgery, radiation, and chemo.

✓ You aren't told that there are natural things you could do to create an environment where cancer won't live (out of the doctor's scope of practice).

✓ Do your research and you'll be ready to incorporate natural alternative methods in conjunction with conventional methods.

✓ Know what you're trying to accomplish with each therapy so you know the results you're looking for (less inflammation, less sugar, less acidity, less pain, shrinking the tumor, stopping tumor growth, balancing the body, etc.).

✓ Don't incorporate a therapy just because someone says it's good. Know why it's good and what it does to the body.

✓ The cells of the body need nutrients. They need to be strong to fight the cancer.

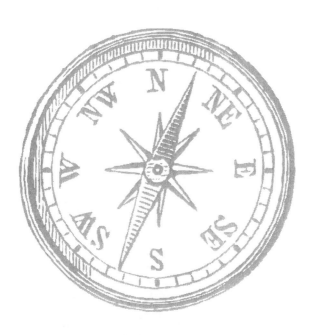

Chapter
NINE

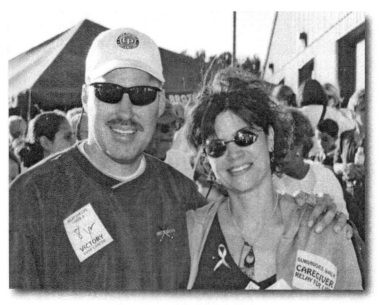

Participating in Relay for Life
American Cancer Society
2006

QUALITY OF LIFE

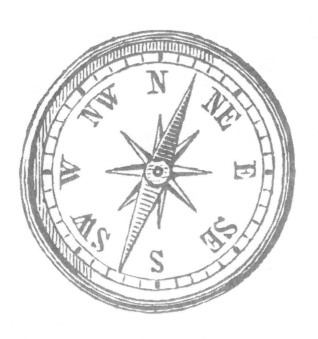

FEBRUARY 2007

⮞ Tommy started acting weird. I called Mary to ask if she could have lunch with him and see if she noticed the same things I did. She met him at his work for lunch on Wednesday. She said she did notice some things that were a bit different and to keep her posted. Thursday, I wouldn't let him go into work because he was having trouble with his speech. He actually argued with me. By that evening, he was better and was helping me cook dinner and wash dishes. We even called Mary and let her talk to him so she could hear that he was doing better.

That night Tommy was up a lot. By around 4:30 in the morning, he was sitting on the side of the bed and got sick. I knew at that point that his brain was swelling. He wasn't able to communicate his issues well. I cleaned him up, got him settled in the bed, and called Mary. We decided to call the oncologist to see if we should go to the emergency room or if they could call in a prescription for Decadron (steroid) to bring down the swelling. The oncologist told us to wait until morning and take him to the hospital to be checked out. After Tommy got sick again I decided to go ahead and take him to the emergency room.

Tommy was able to get up on his own and get into

the car. He kept asking where we were going. By the time we got to the hospital, his balance was off so we had to use a wheelchair. When we checked into the hospital, he couldn't understand what the nurse was asking him. Soon after that, he couldn't speak at all.

He was immediately admitted to the emergency room. Things started moving quickly. I had never seen Tommy change that suddenly. I knew something major was going wrong. I stuck by his side and explained everything to him so he wouldn't be frightened. I also spoke for him to the nursing staff because he couldn't. I began to see fear in his eyes and there was nothing I could do.

Family members began showing up. I got the kids taken care of for the weekend and rearranged the schedule. At that point, I honestly didn't know the full extent of the problem. I was just letting people know where we were and that I would get back to them later. My sister, Kathy, wanted to fly in from Texas. I told her I needed her but that I just didn't know what was going to happen and if it was worth the flight. She decided to come anyway. I was so grateful. Tommy's parents were already on their way to Atlanta from Florida for a regular visit that we had planned earlier. Mary was at the hospital first thing that morning. My parents were there by midmorning. Kim, my sister in California, checked in hourly to get updates and to tell me that she loved me. People were in and out all day.

We quickly got a CAT scan. The neurosurgeon met with Mary and me and told us the scans had shown that the entire left side of Tommy's brain had been taken over by tumor. We weren't prepared to hear that. I was numb. The doctor asked if we had a living will and I said that we did. Was this really it? How long? Oh my God!

Time seemed to be no factor as the day passed. Tommy's body started shutting down hour by hour. His parents made it to the hospital and Tom responded to them. He still couldn't talk and he had lost peripheral vision on the right side. He seemed anxious. Many more friends arrived, so I went to the waiting room to see who was there. Tommy's best friend, Vaughn, came and stayed by my side the rest of the day. It was such a comfort to have him there. The kids were with my parents and had been calling to see how things were going. They knew something was terribly wrong. At that point, I knew I was losing Tommy but I didn't know how fast. I thought we would at least have the weekend.

It was getting late and they finally moved us to a room on a floor. Kathy arrived and we decided to take shifts. Tommy's parents wanted to stay and I had been up since 4:00 a.m. I opted to go to the hotel and get a few hours sleep so that I could be there for the doctor's rounds in the morning.

When Kathy and I got to the hotel, I lost it. I cried so hard. I had never felt this helpless. There was nothing I could do for him. I couldn't bear seeing the fear in his eyes. I eventually fell asleep, but was soon awakened by a phone call from Milton, Tommy's dad. He said that I should come back because Tommy wasn't doing well. I heard a strange sound in the background and asked what it was. At that point the nurse came to the phone. He explained that the sound I heard was Tommy's labored breathing. I hung up the phone and went into panic mode.

Kathy and I threw on our clothes and literally ran down to the car. I made phone calls to Mom and Dad and asked them to bring the kids. They were forty minutes away. I also called Tommy's friend, VT, and my friend, Michele. I don't even know how we got to the hospital, but we did. I jumped out and ran to the room. By that time, Tommy had calmed down and had begun to breathe better. I was relieved but could tell by the look in Milton's eyes that it had been quite an ordeal. We all took a deep breath. That gave us a chance to laugh a little at our escapades to get there, but I vowed I wouldn't leave again.

The nurse came in and asked us to leave the room while they gave Tommy medication rectally due to his being unable to swallow. We all needed a breather so we stepped out into the hall. Vaughn came and gave me a big hug. Mary arrived and was refreshed and ready for a long weekend at the hospital. We joked around with her about that and then went back into the room. As we were putting her things away, Tommy started the weird breathing again. Mary was by his side when he took his last breath. We all quickly surrounded him and watched as the nurse listened for a heartbeat. It was still beating but he wasn't breathing. His heart continued to beat for several minutes. We said tearful, heartfelt, loving goodbyes. Our long fight was over. Tommy was gone.

I cannot put that experience into words. I had no doubt that Tommy's faith was strong but, at the same time, my heart was being ripped out. We were given ample time to be with him and were offered a waiting room. Everything had not sunk in. I was numb and at the same time devastated.

The kids got there about twenty minutes after he had passed. I had to tell them that their father had died. We all hugged and cried. I asked if they wanted to see him. Eric, my middle child who was thirteen, wanted to see him, so I let him. I had no idea what he thought or how it would impact him, but I wanted him to have that option.

I didn't want to be without the kids. I had this overwhelming sense that I needed to protect them. I had to be with them. The kids ended up riding home with me. Kathy drove. It was the longest ride ever. Kathy slept in the bed with me and didn't leave my side.

We only got a few hours of sleep. We had to go to the funeral home that morning which all seemed so surreal. Kim got in early that afternoon and she and Kathy took over things. The house was buzzing with people by the time we returned from the funeral home. The next few days were nonstop. It was all a blur and, as I said, I was totally numb.

The service was actually really good. The kids' school was closed so the students could attend. There was standing room only. Tommy's Navy buddies flew in, which meant a great deal to me. They came to the house and turned up the music. They broke out drinks and celebrated their comrade. Tommy would have loved that. The gesture totally lifted me during such a devastating event. There was nothing like the bond between pilots, especially Navy pilots.

QUALITY OF LIFE

✍ Reflecting back on the events at the hospital, I realized something quite amazing - Tommy had full quality of life all the way till the end. He never had a long, hard struggle. His body literally shut down within twenty-four hours. God took him quickly which was a blessing. The long, determined battle for quality of life was well worth it. We were so blessed to experience Tommy fully all the way until the day he died. We knew he wouldn't grow old with that disease. He had highly malignant brain tumors. However, we were able to experience less brain damage, less sickness, less down time, and more of life because of our efforts.

Some people say that the alternative therapies must not have worked because Tommy didn't make it. I say they worked beautifully. I say they worked better than the traditional treatments of chemo and radiation alone. If you think about it, chemo and radiation didn't work either. They rarely do and, in the process, make your quality of life a living hell!

What is your definition of quality of life? Really, take a moment to think about what that means to you. In my eyes, quality of life is about living life fully. It's about being able to take care of yourself with everyday things such as dressing, eating, and walking. Quality of life is about being a full participant in life. It's about opening presents on Christmas, going to church, volunteering, serving communion, going to cross country meets, and watching your children grow up. It's about going on family trips to the mountains and being able to hike and shop and hang out. It's about going to work and gaining a sense of dignity and pride by contributing to the family. It's about feeling good from the inside out.

Most of the time, it's not the cancer that takes a life - it's the side effects of the treatment. Our goal was to minimize those side effects by combining the treatments. We didn't want Tommy to die prematurely because of a blood clot or organ failure. We were successful in doing just that. Tommy died because the tumors mutated and took over very rapidly. Even if he was on heavy doses of chemotherapy, they would have done the same thing. Tommy died with full quality of life!

Why not combine the two worlds and battle cancer with all you have? Why not lessen the suffering of the side effects? Why not change your lifestyle to prevent the cancer from returning? Why not be an advocate for your own health? It isn't easy, but it's do-able and it's important. Combining treatments makes a difference.

Improving the quality of your life takes a combination of treatments to optimize your results. The idea is to help your body fight the disease. In order to do that, you have to build the immune system. To build the immune system, the body has to recognize and utilize the nutrients you put into it. Doing this, in conjunction with conventional medications, can actually enhance the effects of the drugs and give you a better quality of life.

Here's the Deal:
Why Not Combine the Two Worlds and Battle Cancer with All You Have?

✓ Combining treatments makes a difference!

✓ It helps reduce the suffering and increase the quality of life.

✓ It's not easy, but it's do-able and it's important.

Here's the Deal: Live Life to the Fullest!

✓ What does quality of life mean to you?

✓ In order to feel your best and live life, you have to take on cleaning up your life.

✓ It is so worth the changes required in order to live life to the fullest!

Here's the Deal: It's Up to You and You Alone!

✓ You have to make the decision to incorporate your treatments.

✓ It's your body so you're the one responsible for it.

✓ It's all or nothing. A full life takes full effort. YOU'RE WORTH IT!

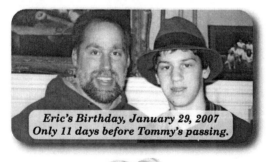

Eric's Birthday, January 29, 2007
Only 11 days before Tommy's passing.

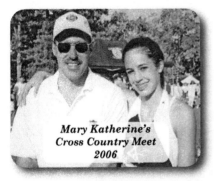

Mary Katherine's Cross Country Meet 2006

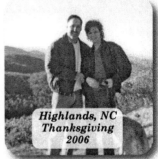

Highlands, NC Thanksgiving 2006

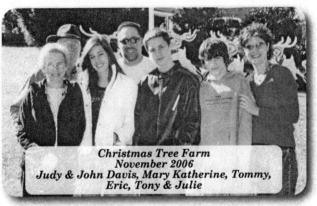

Christmas Tree Farm November 2006 Judy & John Davis, Mary Katherine, Tommy, Eric, Tony & Julie

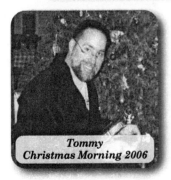

Tommy Christmas Morning 2006

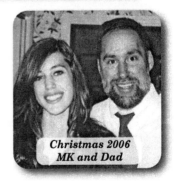

Christmas 2006 MK and Dad

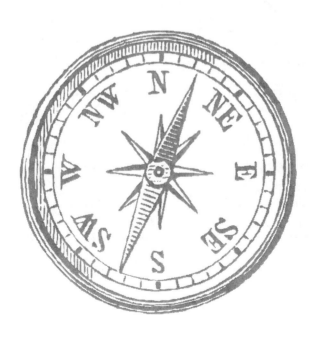

Chapter
TEN

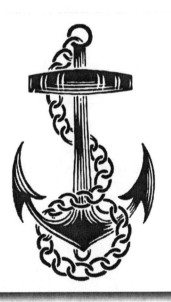

A PASSION TO HELP

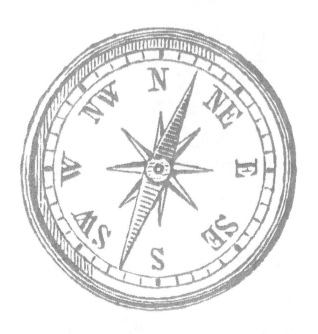

This experience and journey has spoken to my heart. God has placed in me a compassionate desire to help people. It has amazed me that I'm even the least bit interested in the body and how it works. Ten years ago, I would have said you were crazy if you had said that I would be opening up my own practice and helping strangers lessen their suffering. But, that's exactly what I've done.

I completed massage therapy school in July 2007. It was actually a good outlet for me after Tommy's passing. I absolutely loved learning about the body and the hands-on approach. The body is so amazing and the healing powers that each of us has within us is beyond words. I knew I would not stop at basic massage therapy. I already had my sights set on lymphatic drainage. I became more determined than ever to finish my schooling and help people. I passed the national massage therapist certification and started working with a chiropractor. At that point, I really just wanted to increase my massage skills and broaden my experience in the medical field.

After a few months at my first location, I was introduced to a wonderful couple who were physical therapists. They had their own practice and came from a whole body approach. It was a great fit. They helped me find institutes that taught me how to listen to the body in ways I had never experienced. They also allowed me to work with them on patients and have hands-on experience of the therapies. My knowledge and touch expanded. I became more and more passionate about my work and how I could help so many people.

Through multiple continuing education classes and many long weekends away from home, I started gaining certifications and experience that strengthened my understanding and practice. My clients were feeling relief of pain and healing much faster. By incorporating manual therapy from me and a few changes in lifestyle and nutrition, they felt better and were actually amazed that no one had ever told them these things. This gave me such fulfillment and passion to continue my path.

As I took various courses, I realized that I had the most passion for the work centered around cancer patients or chronic illness. I became lymphedema certified so I could work on clients who had lymph nodes removed. I didn't want to hurt my clients in any way and I wanted to work with their doctors to help them heal faster. By getting this certification, both clients and doctors would feel comfortable that I was safe and knew what I was doing.

I focused on lymphatic drainage and oncology massage. The lymph drainage and scar therapies helped cancer clients heal faster and improve their immune function. My clients saw improvement and recovered quicker after only a few sessions. This really got me excited. I knew Tommy always felt so much better after his lymph drainage and massage, but to actually do the work and see the results myself was awesome!

Oncology massage was something I had no idea even existed when I first got into the field. I attended a class and have never looked back. I've attended several more and love the work. It has changed my whole approach to my practice. It's a gift I love giving over and over. The mind and body are so important when healing from a disease. Many times, we disconnect ourselves from the disease. When hands are laid on and an acceptance takes place to meet you just where you are, it's then that the mind and body are brought back together and you can start your healing with power and intent. Oncology massage includes many other aspects of cancer such as scar therapies, lymph drainage, relaxation, and breathing, but the most powerful is just "being in the moment."

When I work on clients with immune issues and disease, their lymph nodes are always congested and thick. I know immediately if the body is fighting something. The major dumping stations are hardened and full. Once I work on them with manual therapy, the nodes dump, the area softens, and the immune system begins to optimally function again. Unfortunately, when fighting a disease, the nodes are working overtime so they don't stay soft and cleared. They tend to fill up which requires weekly treatments to keep them under control. Once in the recovery phase, the treatments can be taken less often until we get into a maintenance phase. I've found that when my clients participate in my lymph program, they are able to tolerate their cancer treatments better, get more sleep, and have an overall better quality of life. The immune function really is so delicate and powerful. Addressing this system helps with your ability to fight disease and feel better.

There is a rather large gap between treatment of cancer and healing of the disease. Chemotherapy, radiation, and surgical treatments can be very invasive, sterile, and cold. Treatment generally takes place in a hospital setting and requires authorizations, referrals, and appointments. Healing, on the other hand, involves rebuilding of the body, which is very noninvasive, warm, and nurturing. Healing takes place in a calm environment without authorizations, referrals, or stressful paperwork. Healing requires rest, time, nurturing, re-growth, acceptance, and empowerment. There needs to be a bridge between treatment and healing. I hope to be that bridge and to assist people with their healing while undergoing treatment.

Many subjects are approached because of my experience with Tommy and the work that I do. Nutrition is still really big in my book. I encourage all my clients to consume raw fruits and vegetables daily and to drink a lot of water. I have found a whole food supplement that is 17 fruits vegetables and grains in capsules. For those that have a hard time eating enough nutrients, I recommend the Juice Plus capsules to bridge that gap. I tell them the benefits of doing so and help them understand the power of food. It's not about the things you don't eat. It's more about the nutrient value that's in the food you do eat. Counting calories and fat isn't the most important thing. Keeping out the chemicals, partially hydrogenated oils, and the denatured foods is more important. Half the battle against disease is nutrition!

Another subject that often comes up is being in tune with your body. It tries to tell you when things are not right, but we dismiss the signs. You really cannot "feel" disease coming on, but you can recognize when you start creating an environment that's optimal for disease growth. Whenever you're exhausted, overly stressed, not eating things with nutrient value (drive-thru food), have chronic digestive issues, are not getting enough sleep, have headaches, allergies, and hormone issues, take a moment and check in with yourself. Don't just look at the isolated condition. Instead, look at what the whole body is telling you. Take a good look at your lifestyle and determine where changes can be made. You would be amazed at how much time and energy you waste on a daily basis. Get back to what is important to you in your life. There's a lot to be said for simple living.

I am no expert in the field of medicine. I appreciate it and respect what it can do for people. Unfortunately, our western society depends on it too much. I actually had a conversation with a 45-year-old friend who said he didn't eat vegetables and would never make small changes like more water and exercise because if something did go wrong there would be a pill to help it. I'm afraid that's the mentality of our culture. You have a headache, take an aspirin. You have a stomachache, take a Tums. Allergies? Pop a Claritin. Get the picture?

Taking care of ourselves isn't "pampering" or a "luxury," - it's a necessity. Tuning into, and becoming aware of your body requires massage therapy, yoga, meditation, prayer, nutrition, and more. It's about slowing down and taking a moment to check in, evaluate, and breathe. Choosing grilled fish and mixed vegetables on a menu isn't about "doing without," it's about nourishing your body and making a better choice. Saying no to someone who asks you to be on a committee or do a project isn't about being selfish, it's about realizing your limits and getting the rest you need to recharge your body. Flip your thinking and re-evaluate your life.

I have had counseling for grief and a lot of advice from friends and family on how to cope with my loss. One of the best exercises I ever did was given by a lady that barely knew me. She merely suggested that I step back and write down everything I loved about Tommy's cancer and my experience with it. I was shocked at her suggestion, but I was willing to try it. I thought it might help me let go of a lot of anger and bitterness toward the illness. This one, soul-searching activity totally changed my perspective and was a great help in getting me through hard times. I want to share my list with you and challenge you to write your own list. You'll soon see the good in everything that happens to you in life.

Things I Love about Cancer/Brain Tumors

- It has defined the meaning of true love.

- It has created family in a way I never thought possible.

- It has shown a man who's a true fighter.

- It has shown a God that is so very real.

- It has given angels in the form of doves.

- It has created a burning desire to help others.

- It has totally changed my outlook on life and what is really important.

- It has given me direction and purpose.

- It has given me something I truly love to do - nutrition.

- It has opened our hearts to the unknown.

- It has built understanding where things were beyond reason.

- It has created strong character in each of us.

- It has taught us to actually play the cards we've been dealt.

- It has revealed the meaning of vulnerability.

- It has developed new friendships where I never thought they existed before.

- It has given hope to others who were scared and overwhelmed.

- It has forced us to go deeper and shed the layers of life and get back to the basics.

- It has taught us not to judge but just to be with others.

- It has humbled us to a point of pure helplessness and trust in the Lord.

- It has opened our minds to new and innovative ideas and shown us a new quality of life.

- It has taught us how to actually make a stand for what we believe no matter what.

- It has created new opportunities to expand our knowledge and lives.

- It has given me the desire to go to massage school and start a new career.

- It has brought us back to Atlanta and closer to family.

- It has helped me develop a better relationship with my parents.

- It has created a trust with my kids that's so very precious.

- It has taught us to accept that life isn't always fair.

- It has developed an acceptance of Tommy no matter what symptoms crop up.

- It has taught us how to cope with unusual circumstances and still smile.

- It has made us stop and acknowledge one another.

- It has helped me overcome and face anger, frustration, and fear.

- It has given us faith, hope, and love.

❧ I don't wish this wake-up call on anyone. However, cancer and degenerative diseases have become an epidemic. Study after study has shown that diet and lifestyle play a large role in both promoting and preventing these diseases. Over 60% of ALL disease could be prevented if we just took better care of ourselves. My journey has revealed a great deal about our bodies, our medical system, and the role we all play in the game of health. Now that I know that drinking more filtered water can prevent colon cancer and arthritis, I'm going to drink it. Now that I know that eating raw foods will prevent the majority of degenerative disease, I'm going to eat them. Now that I know that a stressful lifestyle causes physical damage in the body and creates an environment in which cancer can grow, I'll slow down and find ways to relieve the stress and become more balanced.

My life will never be the same after this journey. I'll always have an incredible passion to help others make their own lives nothing short of extraordinary.

When I was a kid, one of my favorite shows was Let's Make A Deal. I was always fascinated by what might be behind the various curtains and doors. The thought of the contestants making the wrong choice made me a nervous wreck! But it was the best when, after going back and forth as to what to do, they made their choice and won something really fantastic, like a new car. Do you remember that show?

Through this book, I wanted to let you peek behind the curtains, look inside the boxes, and encourage you to begin seriously thinking about which choices could pay off for you big time and warn you about the choices that could cost you EVERYTHING. In short, I wanted you to know the right choices before you were forced to make the biggest deal of your life. Please - choose wisely.

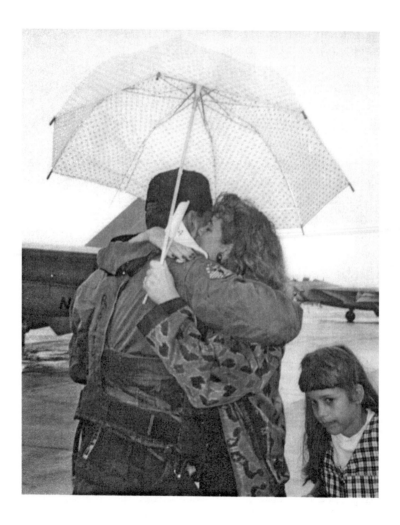

References

Batmanghelidj, F. 2008. *Your Body's Many Cries for Water.* Falls Church: Global Health Solutions, Inc.

Campbell, T. Colin. 2006. The China Study: The Most Comprehensive Study of Nutrition Ever Conducted and the Startling Implications for Diet, Weight Loss and Long-term Health. Dallas: Benbella Books.

Harter Pierce, T. 2009. *Outsmart Your Cancer: Alternative Non-toxic Treatments that Work.* Stateline: Thoughtworks Publishing.

Popper, Pamela A. *The Wellness Forum: Wellness 101.* Worthington: The Wellness Forum Center.

Popper, Pamela A. *The Wellness Forum: Wellness 201, Text for Level Two Certification.* Worthington: The Wellness Forum Center.

Santillo, Humbart. 1993. *Food Enzymes: Missing Link to Radiant Health.* Twin Lakes: Lotus Press.

Somers, Suzanne. 2010. *Knockout: Interviews with Doctors Who Are Curing Cancer—and How to Prevent Getting It in the First Place.* New York: Three Rivers Press.

Trudeau, Kevin. 2006. *Natural Cures "They" Don't Want You To Know About.* Birmingham: Alliance Publishing Group.

Resources

American Cancer Society (Information)
http://www.cancer.org/

Antioxidants and Free Radicals
Nutri Team
Dr. Richard Dubois, NSA
http://www.nutriteam.com/antiox.htm

Body of Health
Julie D. Mills, CMT, LLCC (Author and Therapist)
www.bodyofhealthandlife.com
Email: Julie@bodyofhealthandlife.com

The Cancer Cure Foundation (Information)
http://www.cancure.org/

Cancer Tutor
http://www.cancertutor.com/Cancer/Protocel.html

Chikly Health Institute
(Directory and Education)
Lymph Drainage Therapy
http://www.chiklyinstitute.org/

Far Infrared Therapy
http://www.firheals.com/catalog/far_infrared_therapy.php

Glycemic Index
http://www.glycemicindex.com/

The Herring Foundation of Hope
(Hope Kit and Education)
http://www.herringhope.org/

Hospital Santa Monica (Treatment & Detox)
(Donsbach Clinic)
Rosarita Beach, Mexico
Run by Dr. Kurt Donsbach, DC, ND, PhD
http://www.donsbach.com
Phone: 800-359-6547 or 619-427-3007

IMMUNE RECOVERY CENTERS OF AMERICA
(Treatment & Detox)
4536 Chamblee Dunwoody Rd., Ste. 250
Dunwoody, GA 30338
Ph: 770-455-6100 Fax: 770-455-1999
www.immunerecovery.net

Insulin Potentiaion Therapy
http://www.immunerecovery.net/IPT%20History.htm

Juice Plus+ (Whole Food in Capsules)
https://www.bodyofhealthandlife.com

Life Extension (Supplements)
http://www.lef.org/

National Cancer Institute (Information)
http://www.cancer.gov

National Institutes of Health (Information)
http://www.nih.gov/

Nutritional Solutions
(Nutritionist/Supplements)
Jeanne M. Wallace, PhD, CNC
1697 East, 3450 North
North Logan, Utah 84341 USA
(435) 563-0053
Email: admin@nutritional-solutions.ne
http://www.nutritional-solutions.net/

Moss Reports (Information)
Ralph W. Moss, PhD
http://www.cancerdecisions.com/

Protocel (Supplement/Treatment)
http://www.outsmartyourcancer.com/ebooklet.asp

Raw Food Made Easy (Recipes)
Jennifer Cornbleet
www.learnrawfood.com

Rife Machines
http://www.rife.org/
Read more at:
http://www.ehow.com/how-does_5063622_rife-machines-work.html#ixzz0znRU2cTi

Dr. Smokey Santillo (Author/Doctor/Whole Body)
http://www.smokeysantillo.com/

Society for Oncology Massage (Directory of Therapists/Education)
http://www.s4om.org/div1/index.htm

Touch For Health (Education)
Whole Body Balancing and Therapy
http://www.tfhka.org/

Otto Warburg
Prime Cause and Prevention of Cancer
http://new-planet.net/pdf/O-Warburg-CancerProtocol.pdf

The Wellness Forum (Courses and Counseling)
Pam Popper, PhD, ND
http://www.wellnessforum.com

Did you know...?

▶ Eating 6 servings per day of fruits and vegetables cuts the stroke rate by 44%.

▶ Eating 9 servings per day of fruits and vegetables cuts the stroke rate by 66%.

▶ Apples have natural estrogen and help reduce cholesterol.

▶ Acerola cherries are known to relieve symptoms of osteoarthritis.

▶ Raw beets are a natural antidepressant.

▶ Blueberries lower cholesterol better than drugs.

▶ Broccoli is a super source of chromium, which helps regulate insulin and blood sugar, and it has 20-50% more anti-cancer capabilities than Tamoxifin.

▶ Cabbage is anti-ulcer, and eating Cabbage more than once per week cuts colon cancer odds by 66%.

▶ Carrots fight heart and eye disease, and eating a Carrot a day cuts the stroke rate in women by 68%.

▶ Cranberries are strong antibiotics and antivirals.

▶ Kale has 50% more calcium than milk.

▶ Oranges, besides being high in vitamin C, have every class of cancer inhibitor known.

▶ Papayas are natural medicine for helping digestion.

▶ Parsley lowers blood pressure.

▶ Peaches contain Boron, which aids in Calcium absorption.

▶ Pineapple is your best anti-inflammatory and helps dissolve blood clots.

▶ Eating a half cup of spinach once a day cuts macular degeneration odds by 43%, and it lowers cholesterol.

▶ Tomatoes reduce your risk of skin, pancreatic, bladder, and prostate cancer.

Did you know that all these fruits and vegetables are also your best source of antioxidants to protect from degenerative diseases such as cancer, heart disease, and diabetes?

Food Tips

- Get creative with your salads. It's important to get a variety of vegetables into your daily routine. A good way to do that is with salads. If you're not fond of a particular vegetable you can grate it, shred it, or tear off small pieces to blend into a salad with little taste but a lot of nutrition.

Remember, raw vegetables can be delicious in and of themselves. Try to enhance the flavor with mild spices instead of covering up the fresh taste of the food.

Salad Ingredients:

- Romaine lettuce
- Spinach leaves
- Chopped carrots
- Chopped cucumbers
- Thinly sliced red cabbage
- Grated yellow squash
- Grated zucchini
- Sliced tomatoes
- Alfalfa sprouts (very little taste but packed with nutrition)

You can always add grilled salmon or chicken on top to make a full meal. For salad dressing I recommend Newman's Own brand. I prefer to stay with the oil and vinegar dressing and keep it as simple as possible.

- Cut up raw vegetables and serve with ranch dressing. (Use Newman's Own because it has no MSG.)

- Keep boiled eggs on hand. They fill you up, add flavor, and they're easy. Add to salads, eat for breakfast, or as a snack.

- Raw nuts (walnuts, almonds, sunflower seeds, soy nuts) fill you up, provide Omega-3, and they're easy.

- How to cook green beans or asparagus:
  Cut off the tips of green beans or the ends of asparagus. Put the vegetables in a frying pan. Cut off two tablespoons butter (not margarine) and put on stack of beans or asparagus. Cut half a lime into wedges and squeeze over veggies and put the other half in the pan. Squirt 2-3 tablespoons of Braggs Amino over the veggies. Simmer for 5-10 minutes (heated but still crunchy).

- Put the following in a dish or baggie to marinate before cooking:

  - Grilled Chicken/Meats:

- Newman's Own Vinaigrette
- Braggs Amino
- Red wine (optional)

- Have all natural almond butter and whole wheat sprouted bread (Ezekiel) on hand for snacks or lunch option.

- Wraps are great to make beforehand and have ready to go. Combine fresh spinach, sprouts, deli meat, and Swiss cheese with a dab of balsamic vinaigrette and you have a healthy meal to go. Slice up an apple and add a few Joseph's cookies and that's a meal. Note: 1) Use whole wheat tortillas without partially hydrogenated oils. Read the label when choosing a wrap—spinach, whole wheat, plain—and make sure it doesn't contain shortening or hydrogenated oils. 2) Many deli meats contain preservatives and nitrates. Look for all-natural brands such as Applegate, Plainsville, and Boar's Head Oven Gold Turkey.)

- Another idea for wraps (good hot or cold and great for on-the-go):

  - 1 can black beans drained
  - 1/4 cup salsa
  - Grated cheddar cheese
  - Couscous (optional)

- Corn chips and salsa makes a good snack as well.

- Stay away from fried foods. Order grilled when eating out. Opt for the salad or grilled veggies instead of the potato.

- Use a wok to heat up leftovers or just to throw together a few veggies for lunch. You can always put a spoonful of salsa into anything to add flavor.

- I recommend cooking up a pot of brown rice to use throughout the week. It takes 40-60 min. to cook so cooking a lot at once will save time.

- Drink your coffee if need be, but drink a full glass of water before the coffee to cut down on acidity. You might want to drink hot green tea instead of coffee. It's good for you and still warm.

- Water, water, water is your best bet. At least a gallon a day! Gulp it, don't sip it.

- Prepare Juice Plus Complete shakes in the mornings. Recipe:

  - One scoop of Juice Plus Complete powder
  - 1 c. strawberries
  - 1 banana

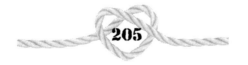

- 1 cup Spinach
- 1 carrot
- 1 c. soy, rice, or almond milk
- ½ c. orange juice
- 1 c. ice

Place in blender and mix. Add additional milk for desired consistency. Add blueberries, blackberries, pineapple, melon, or whatever fruit or vegetables you have on hand.

Food List

Things to have on hand in your pantry:

Basil
Black beans - canned
Braggs Amino Acids (instead of soy sauce)
Chick peas - canned
Chopped tomatoes - canned
Couscous (found in the rice section)
Cumin
Extra virgin organic olive oil
Garlic powder
Garlic salt
Lime juice
Minced garlic
Minced onion
Newman's Own Balsamic Vinaigrette
Oregano
Organic tomato sauce - canned
Pepper

Raw honey
Rice Dream Milk (instead of regular milk)
Sea Salt
Simply Orange orange juice (not from concentrate)
  - Tropicana orange juice will do if you can't find Simply Orange
Soy milk for your shakes
Stevia (instead of sugar)
Vinegar (preferably apple cider or balsamic)
Whole wheat pastas
Brown Rice
Oatmeal
Lentils

Fresh Fruits:
  Apples
  Strawberries
  Blueberries
  Bananas - these are high in sugar so just a few
  (Note: fruit has sugar, so limit it to just a few servings a day or to flavor something)

Fresh Vegetables:
  Bell peppers
  Onions
  Garlic
  Sweet potatoes
  Zucchini
  Squash
  Sprouts—alfalfa, clover, bean—they're packed full of nutrients in salads or on sandwiches

Spinach
Romaine lettuce
Tomatoes
Carrots
Purple cabbage—put in salads. It has very little
taste but a lot of nutrients.

That should get you started. Don't buy in bulk.
You'll have to go to the grocery store more than
once a week because fresh foods go bad quickly.
There are no preservatives anymore! I realize this
is an adjustment, but like exercise, you will get
used to it.

Tommy's Chicken Soup

This chicken soup recipe was Tommy's favorite.
When he was going through chemo this was the
only thing he could keep down. I believe the broth
and fennel soothed his stomach and helped him feel
better. The soup is healthier because it doesn't have
any additives or preservatives. It's simple and
made with TLC.

Ingredients:
    1 whole range-free chicken (about 3-4 lbs.)
    1 medium onion, quartered
    1 bunch celery (cut off bottom and clean stalks)
    3 tablespoons fennel seed
    2 tablespoons sea salt

1 teaspoon pepper
2 tablespoons ketchup
2 cups Private Select Acini Di Pepe pasta or small star noodles.

Directions:
Fill large boiling pot (6 qt.) 2/3 full with water (4 qt.) Add chicken, onion, celery, fennel, salt, and pepper. Bring to a boil for 10 minutes. Lower heat and simmer 3 hours or until chicken starts to fall off the bone.

Place another large boiling pot in the sink and put a colander in the pot. Dump the cooked soup into the colander over large pot (you are separating broth). Let cool about 10-15 minutes. Lift out the colander full of chicken and vegetables, hold to drain over the pot and place onto a plate. With a fork, pick the meat off the chicken bones and put back into the pot of broth. Throw away the bones and all that is in the colander.

Return the broth to the stove and bring to a boil. Add 2 cup private select Acini Di Pepe pasta or any small noodles to the boiling broth. Cook for 25 minutes. Add ketchup. Stir well and serve.

Herring Foundation
Quick Start Guide to Cancer

So you or someone you care about has cancer. After the initial shock of hearing that word you realize it's time to get down to business and beat this disease. This Guide is a tool to help you get started doing just that.

First, take a deep breath. Clear your mind of any preconceived notions you have about cancer and its treatment. Then read the guide. Take notes, do some research, make a plan, and then get started implementing that plan. The following is a step-by-step guide written by people just like you. We, too, were in your shoes and didn't know where to start after hearing the words cancer, malignant, surgery, chemotherapy, radiation. You feel the blood rushing and beating in your ears because it's just too much to take in. Well, now that you are ready, here is a kick-start guide. It is based on real life experience and what we have learned in our journey through cancer and its treatment.

1. Do NOT Panic

First and foremost, DO NOT PANIC! There are people who are living with cancer or as cancer survivors. While you may feel rushed to make a decision yesterday, it's okay to give yourself a little time to breath and take it all in. It's important that YOU take control of this situation and your health. Take a minute or two to wallow in your diagnosis but then shake it off and refocus your life. Yes, your life has just changed tracks unexpectedly and that can be quite shocking. But it is what it is and now is the time to refocus and take command of this train known as your life and your health.

The cancer didn't develop overnight. It took time to grow and while it's important that you start treating your cancer quickly you do have some time to make a plan and the only plan worth following is a well-informed plan. No, you might not have all the answers because you did not go to medical school but you DO have access to more information than you realize. Let's tap into that information so you can make the MOST informed decisions possible for your health right now. You can make adjustments as you learn more and as your situation evolves. YOU are in control!

2. Educate Yourself; Know your Disease

It's important that you learn as much as you can about your type of cancer and how cancer was able to grow in your body. If you are unable to or do not want to do a lot of research, choose someone from your support group to be your lead researcher. No matter who you choose you need this person to be organized, articulate and as objective as possible. It should be someone you respect and can work with.

Your researchers should search the web for your type of cancer. Find a discussion group or listserve to determine which hospitals and research facilities are at the top of the field for your particular type of cancer. It is important that you be informed on how your cancer forms and exactly where it is. For example, brain tumors are hard to treat because the brain has a blood/brain barrier to protect it. Many medications and treatments cannot penetrate the blood/brain barrier and are therefore ineffective. Find out about your particular type of cancer and its location so you can make the best decision regarding your treatment. Find other people with your type of cancer and learn what has and has not worked for them.

It's important to know and understand what type of environment was going on in your body that allowed the cancer cells to develop and grow. With this understanding, you can make a better, and more informed, decision on how you plan to tackle your treatment.

Remember, information and knowledge are power!

3. Be Open to All Options

While you may choose a treatment that is specific to your type of cancer, it is imperative that you treat the WHOLE body. The body cannot be isolated. Each part has its role in maintaining or undermining optimum health and therefore needs to be treated wholly in order to regain that balance of optimum health. There are a myriad of treatments available. Be open to many different types. It may be that you find an integrative approach works best. Be open to what comes your way. Try to let go of preconceived notions so you can make the most informed choice you can make.

Think of filling a toolbox with the best cancer-fighting and body-building tools you can find. Here are some items you need in your toolbox (This is a generic list of potential tools. You will need to fill in the specifics): Medical team, treatment plan, alternative practitioners (massage therapy, lymphatics, acupuncture, nutritional consultants, etc.), family and friends, food, supplements, exercise, other cancer survivors and/or caregivers.

4. Choose your Cancer-fighting Team; You Are Director of the Board

Once you've done your initial research you will need to choose your medical team. Appoint someone to be your CEO. Think of your team as the "We are going to beat cancer" corporation. You are the

Director of the Board. Ultimately it is you who has control over your health and your healthcare. Make sure you build a good team around you in order to succeed. Your CEO will guide and direct your team. (If the CEO is other than the patient it should be someone trusted and respected by the patient.)

It's important to believe in and trust your medical team. It is okay to go to another doctor that specializes in your type of cancer. Your local doctors are doing the best they can with what they have access to. Look for research hospitals that have the new trials and equipment. This is why it is important to get online with chat groups and ask people with your type cancer where they are going. Take that information and look to see how many patients they see on average with your type cancer. If it is only a few, keep looking. If it is hundreds, bingo! If you aren't sure about a doctor or healthcare provider go to another for a second or third opinion. Make sure you are comfortable with that doctor and that he/she fits into your plan for your treatment.

5. Choose Treatment

Now that you have your information and your medical team it's time to decide how you are going to treat your cancer. Listen to your team, look at your research, and then make a decision and move forward. Whether you choose to go with a conventional-only plan, an alternative-only plan, or an integrated approach it is important that you know YOU are in control. Take responsibility for your health in ALL aspects. Find out what else you can do to help your body heal itself. There are options out there from nutrition and supplements to massage and lymph therapies as well as acupuncture, etc., that can help you as you help your body heal.

Set a goal and a time frame to reassess (possibly after every scan which is about every two months). What you are looking for is tumor status and quality of life status. Is the tumor the same or no growth, shrinking, or growing? Am I able to participate in life? (Some discomfort is inevitable, but you do not have to be bedridden! This is where the alternative is so important.) At some point in time, you will have to go with a choice based on the information you have.

6. Importance of Diet, Nutrition, and Supplements

Our bodies are designed to heal themselves. Think about how a cut heals itself in a week's time. That's how we work on the inside as well. Cancer is a mutation of cells. We all have cancer cells in our bodies but those of us with intact immune systems can fight off the cells before they can grow and spread. In order to give your body the tools it needs to heal itself you must give it the proper nutrients. A plant-based, whole food, whole grain approach is best. Avoid chemicals and processed foods that can actually damage our bodies on the cellular level and sometimes create an environment that allows cancer to flourish. If you eat animal proteins choose lean, minimally processed meats and fish. The following information is research describing the link between diet and cancer.

The link between diet and cancer is not new. The January 1892, Scientific American printed the observation that "cancer is most frequent among those branches of the human race where carnivorous habits prevail." Numerous research studies have shown that cancer is much more common in populations consuming diets rich in fatty foods, particularly meat, and much less common in countries eating diets rich in grains, vegetables, and fruits. One reason is that foods affect the action of hormones in the body. They also affect the strength of the immune system and other factors. While fruits and vegetables contain a variety of vitamins, minerals, antioxidants, and phytochemicals to protect the body, by contrast, recent research shows that animal products contain potentially carcinogenic compounds which may contribute to increased cancer risk.[1]

[1]Skog KI, Johansson MAE, Jagerstad MI. Carcinogenic heterocyclic amines in model systems and cooked foods: a review on formation, occurrence, and intake. Food and Chem Toxicol 1998; 36:879-96.

The Cancer Recovery Foundation has the following to say about diet and cancer:

- 30-40% of cancers are directly related to dietary habits.

- Obesity is one of the major risk factors for developing cancer and it has a negative effect on treatment outcomes.

- Divide your dinner plate: 2/3 or more of the plate for vegetables, fruits, whole grains and beans, 1/3 or less for animal protein.

- Phytonutrients such as flavonoids, carotenoids, and lycopene may help fight against cancer. The different color of the fruits and vegetables give you different phytonutrients. The darker the color, the more nutrient value. Almost all fruits and vegetables are good sources of these nutrients. A variety of color is the most effective way to get a good variety of nutrients.

- Include sources of omega-3 oils, such as fatty fish, canola oil, flax seeds, or flax seed oils and walnuts.

- About 30% of cancer deaths are caused by malnutrition and not the cancer. Adequate nutrition before, during, and after treatment is important! Your body will need adequate calories, protein, vitamins, and minerals.

- Some types of cancers cause increased metabolism (the body burns more calories than it normally would) which can lead to general weight loss and/or muscle wasting.

- Proper nutrition will help your body fight against cancer and cope better with treatments.

- Well-nourished people may recuperate faster after treatments are finished and even be able to tolerate higher amounts of treatments. Frequent small meals can be easier to tolerate and more appealing than three larger meals, so you might want to eat every 2 to 3 hours.

- When you are not consuming enough nutritious foods your body will use its nutrient stores for energy. This may weaken your immunity and ability to fight infection and other assaults on your body.

- If you are unable to meet your nutritional requirements due to poor appetite or difficulty eating caused by treatment side effects, you may benefit from nutritional (whole food) supplements. These come as drinks or shakes, powders and puddings, and can be purchased from most supermarkets and pharmacies. Try them chilled and in different flavors. Discuss your need for supplements with your doctor or a registered dietician. (Just get the nutrients in. Try juicing, vita mix, or blending veggies, etc.) Use as many whole food supplements as possible, not fragmented, isolated vitamins. At this point in your recovery, the body needs every enzyme, fiber, phyto-nutrient, and mineral from the whole plant.

- Water is the most essential element, next to air, for our survival. Water is everywhere, yet most people take it for granted. Water makes up more than two thirds of our weight. Our brain, blood, and lungs consist mostly of water.

- Blood is 83% water

- Muscles are 75% water

- The brain is 74% water

- Bone is 22% water

Even a slight 2% drop in our body's water supply can cause us to show signs of dehydration.

- Dry mouth and tongue with thick saliva
- Flushed face
- Dry, warm skin
- Dizziness
- Weakness
- Muscle cramps
- Sleepy
- Irritable
- Headaches

Mild dehydration is one of the most common causes of daytime fatigue. An estimated seventy-five percent of Americans have mild, chronic dehydration. This is hard to believe where water is readily available through the tap or bottle.

Adapted from Cancer Resource by American Institute for Cancer Research

7. Attitude (Support and Spirituality)

Our thoughts can sometimes make us sick. Explore various avenues with which you are comfortable to nurture your spirituality. It's important to find a few minutes each day to sit in quiet and peace whether you are praying or just taking solace in a few minutes of tranquility.

According to Robert Moss, "Scientists first proved a link between stress and disease in the early half of the last century. Since then, researchers have examined old and new practices including biofeedback, meditation, guided imagery, spiritual healing, and deep breathing. The fast-expanding field of psychoneuroimmunology, which examines how the neurological and immune systems interact, is providing new clinical evidence of the connection between thoughts and health."

8. Exercise

Exercise is very important for the cancer patient. Studies have shown how important it is for health and wellness. Kim Walker, a cancer exercise specialist at the Huntsman Cancer Institute in Salt Lake City, seeing how exercise helped cancer patients minimize fatigue and depression, had the following to say about cancer and exercise: "Many patients in treatment feel as if 'my life's not my own,'. Exercising gives them a sense of control. It's empowering."

Dr. Theodore Pollock practices at Cancer Treatment Centers of America at Southwestern Regional Medical Center in Tulsa, Oklahoma[2]. He says exercise is good for overall health, but he states: "There's enough data now to show that people who are physically active do better, they respond to

treatment better, they experience less toxicity and in some cases, they live longer."
[2]Dallas Morning News

Please seek the advice of your medical team before starting an exercise program. It's important to have exercise in your arsenal of cancer fighting tools!

9. Review and Recap

- Take a deep breath
- Decide to fight cancer
- Build your team and your toolbox
- Give your body the nutrients/tools it needs to fight the cancer
- Get moving
- Reduce your stress
- Create a positive attitude and develop your spiritual being

My Favorite Quote

"Our deepest fear is not that we are inadequate. Our deepest fear is that we are powerful beyond measure. It is our light, not our darkness that most

frightens us. We ask ourselves, 'Who am I to be brilliant, gorgeous, talented, fabulous?' Actually, who are you not to be? You are a child of God. Your playing small does not serve the world. There is nothing enlightened about shrinking so that other people won't feel insecure around you. We are all meant to shine, as children do. We were born to make manifest the glory of God that is within us. It's not just in some of us; it's in everyone. And as we let our own light shine, we unconsciously give other people permission to do the same. As we are liberated from our own fear, our presence automatically liberates others." Our Deepest Fear
by Marianne Williamson from A Return To Love: Reflections on the Principles of A Course in Miracles

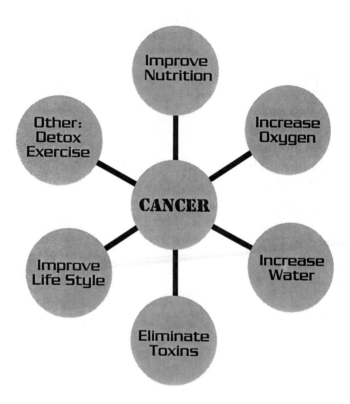

Caner does not stem from one thing; it is an environment in which you create. Incorporating all of the above will help create a healthy environment for the body to fight disease.

Appendix

Alkaline Foods		Acid Foods	
Vegetables Asparagus Artichokes Cabbage Lettuce Onion Cauliflower Radish Swede Lambs Lettuce Peas Courgette Red Cabbage Leeks Watercress Spinach Turnip Chives Carrot Green Beans Beetroot Garlic Celery Grasses (wheat, straw, barley, dog, kamut etc.) Cucumber Broccoli Kale Brussels Sprouts	**Fruits** Lemon Lime Avocado Tomato Grapefruit Watermelon (is neutral) Rhubarb **Drinks** 'Green Drinks' Fresh vegetable juice Pure water (distilled or ionized) Lemon water (pure water + fresh lemon or lime). Herbal Tea Vegetable broth Non-sweetened Soy Milk Almond Milk **Seeds, Nuts & Grains** Almonds Pumpkin Sunflower Sesame Flax Buckwheat Groats Spelt Lentils Cumin Seeds Any sprouted seed	**Meats** Pork Lamb Beef Chicken Turkey Crustaceans Other Seafood (apart from occasional oily fish such as salmon) **Others** Vinegar White Pasta White Bread Wholemeal Bread Biscuits Soy Sauce Tamari Condiments (Tomato Sauce, Mayonnaise etc.) Artificial Sweeteners Honey **Convenience Foods** Sweets Chocolate Microwave Meals Tinned Foods Powdered Soups Instant Meals Fast Food	**Dairy Products** Milk Eggs Cheese Cream Yogurt Ice Cream **Drinks** Fizzy Drinks Coffee Tea Beers Spirits Fruit Juice Dairy Smoothies Milk Traditional Tea **Fats & Oils** Saturated Fats Hydrogenated Oils Margarine (worse than Butter) Corn Oil Vegetable Oil Sunflower Oil
Fats & Oils Flax Hemp Avocado Olive Evening Primrose Borage Coconut Oil Oil Blends (such as Udo's Choice)	**Others** Sprouts (soy, alfalfa, mung bean, wheat, little radish, chickpea, broccoli etc) Bragg Liquid Aminos (Soy Sauce Alternative) Hummus Tahini	**Fruits** All fruits aside from those listed in the alkaline column.	**Seeds & Nuts** Peanuts Cashew Nuts Pistachio Nuts

General Guidance:
Stick to salads, fresh vegetables, healthy nuts, and oils. Try to consume plenty of raw foods and at least 2-3 liters of clean, pure water daily (ideally enhanced with pH drops).

General Guidance:
Steer clear of fatty meats, dairy, cheese, sweets, chocolate, alcohol, and tobacco. Packaged foods are often full of hidden offenders and microwave meals are full of sugars and salts. Overcooking removes the nutrition from a meal!

CPSIA information can be obtained at www.ICGtesting.com
Printed in the USA
LVOW11s0620211013

357763LV00001B/2/P

9 780986 015915